AGRICULTURAL ENVIRONMENT AND HEALTH

About the Author

S. Waseem, A. Ashraf (*b.* 1952) is a faculty in Geography at the Aligarh Muslim University, Aligarh. Earlier, he served in different teaching and non-teaching capacities abroad. His field of specialization is Environmental, Agricultural and Medical Geography. Dr. Ashraf has published many research papers in national and international journals of repute.

AGRICULTURAL ENVIRONMENT AND HEALTH

Dr. S.Waseem A. Ashraf

CONCEPT PUBLISHING COMPANY, NEW DELHI-110059

Cataloging in Publication Data—DK
Courtesy: D.K. Agencies (P) Ltd. <docinfo@dkagencies.com>

Ashraf, S. Waseem A., 1952-
Agricultural environment and health / S. Waseem A. Ashraf.
p. cm.
Study conducted at Central Ganga-Ghagra Doab area of Uttar Pradesh and Uttaranchal states of India.
Includes bibliographical references (p.)
Includes index.
ISBN 818069304X

1. Agricultue—Environmental aspects—India—Ganges-Ghagra Doab. 2. Environmental health—India—Ganges-Ghagra Doab. I. Title.

DDC 362.109 54 22

ISBN : 81-8069-304-X

First Published 2006

Published and Printed by
Ashok Kumar Mittal
Concept Publishing Company
A/15-16, Commercial Block, Mohan Garden,
New Delhi-110059 (India)

Phones : 25351460, 25351794
Fax : +91-11-25357103
Email : publishing@conceptpub.com

Dedicated

to

My Parents

Acknowledgements

I take this opportunity to express my deep sense of gratitude to (late) Dr. Niaz Ahmad Siddiqi who was on the teaching faculty of the department of Geography and who helped immensely in the completion of this work and without his active assistance the work would not have seen the light of the day.

I am also thankful to the Chairman of the Department of Geography for providing necessary facilities in the completion of this work.

My sincere thanks are due to Laureat d' Honneur (IGU) and Bhoogol Ratna Professor Emeritus Dr. Mohammad Shafi my esteemed teacher for his inspiration, guidance and encouragement in the completion of this work.

I would be failing in my duty if I do not express my sincere thanks to my colleagues, particularly Prof. Ali Mohammad, Dr. Abdul Munir for going through the manuscript and for providing valuable suggestions and comments.

Dr. Hifzur Rahman and Dr. Farasat Ali Siddiqi on the teaching staff of the Department were kind enough to extend their help whenever I needed it. I should also thank Computer Section of the Department as well as the office personnel in helping me to complete this work.

Contents

List of Tables

List of Maps

List of Maps

1 Introduction

In the study of human nutrition, geography occupies as important a position as any other branch of life science. Nutrition has assumed so much significance in the present era that its study becomes important in maintaining good health and preserving the body from the ill effects of communicable and deficiency diseases. Hence, the aim of this study is to critically examine the nutrients and the quantity that should be supplied to human body for normal growth and protection from ailments. This depends very much on the nature of food produced and its proper distribution. The question may arise as to what type of food should be produced that has nutritive value and what method of distribution should be adopted so that it could be within easy reach of each individual. In the present socio-economic condition it is not easy for the farmers to realize the importance of those food crops which have sufficient quantity of nutrition. Whatever food is produced in the country, its major portion is consumed locally. The rich get richer, and the poor get poorer. Even with the Green Revolution there is continued under-nutrition situation in some areas. Nutrition scarcity areas do not get sufficient supply from the good nutritionally productive areas. This phenomenon causes great hindrance in the way of maintaining good health. Further, the dietary habits of the rural population are determined by the physical and social environment factors and their food lacks nutritive value.

However, in recent years some awakening with regard to changes in the nature of food supply, dietary habits and standard of living is witnessed among the rural communities. Once the benefits that accrue from nutritive diets are known to the farming community a change for better health programme is bound to take place. The rural development schemes envisaged by the governments, will surely go a long way in educating the village people about the value of nutritive diets and good health.

It is axiomatic that the destiny of a nation lies more in healthy population, but many of us rarely appreciate the fact that a vast majority of our population is ill-fed, ill-clad, and live in dilapidated houses. The vicious circle of disease low production – low income – poor health services – more disease and more poverty not only poses a problem of health and sanitation but also of social welfare and social justice[1].

Mal-nutrition is one of the most important health problems of the country. It is estimated that about 70 per cent of the country's population suffers from mal and under-nutrition. This is the result of either of chronic insufficiency of food or of inadequacy of the protective foods necessary for a healthy life or a combination of both. Thus, general hunger or hunger for specific essential nutrients produces adverse effects which are of far reaching nature.

Infants born of mal-nourished mothers start life with a handicap. In a few months or a year, many of them die of mal-nutrition alone or due to mal-nourishment they succumb easily to gastro-intestinal and respiratory infections. The prevalence of various communicable diseases in the areas of hunger and mal-nutrition makes situation still more serious. In identifying deficiency diseases, there are a number of factors to examine at children level. Deficiency of protein if it occurs in children up to the age of 5 years is bound to produce some deficiency deceases. Similarly in deficiency of vitamins-A, C and D leave to a number of deficiency diseases.

Kwashirkor's – a Ghanan word most obvious symptoms are complete wasting away of the child. Their limbs aren't much larger than the bones underneath the skin. Often, their bellies are huge and protruding. This is called 'pot belly' and their facial feature are pale and depressed. Anyone can recognize this in a child suffering from Kwashirkor. A total lack of anyone of the many important nutrients will cause illness, and eventually death, if the deficiency persist for a long period of time. That is why the nutrients called "essential nutrients".

The area under study lies in the eastern Uttar Pradesh, comprising the districts of Faizabad, Ambedkar Nagar[2] and Sultanpur situated in the Central Ganga-Ghaghara Doab. This area is relatively less developed in the spheres of industries, agriculture, health and urbanization. Areas like this have dual disadvantage of heavy population and low food supply. Lack of jobs and low purchasing power have reduced the accessibility of nutrient food causing many deficiencies. Poverty is also hindrance in the protection of the environment. Dilapidated houses restrict fresh air, non-availability of pure drinking water, non-accessibility of nutrient food are some of the major causes of deficiency deceases.

In the study of human nutrition, inter-disciplinary approaches have made a successful progress. However, Geographers have studied human health problems by undertaking distributional pattern of deceases. The study of environmental factors the geography occupies an important position. The study of human health problems and environment comes under the recently introduced specialized branch of geography, i.e. "Medical Geography". The term was first coined though by non-geographers like Leonhard, Ludwig Finke, but Jacques May took the subject matter further in a systematic way by taking physical, cultural factors along with pathological factors as a determinant of human health. Also the study of environmental factors which ought to have influence the human health have been studied by McGlashan (1969). According to Pyle (1979) ecological approach to studies of the Geography of human illness is considered by many in Medical Geography and the temporary recognition to the branch accorded in the IGU (International Geographical Union) at Lisbon, to define the Medical Geography and understanding medical ecology. In its report of Medical Geography was defined as the study, of geographical factors concerned with cause and effects of health and disease. The permanent status to this field of specialization was granted only in 1968 IGU under the chairmanship of A.T.A. Learmonth. Environment was always the core for the geographers to study health.

Although systematic study of the subject is going on for last five decades but the essence could be traced back in ancient study e.g. in essay on air, water, place by Hippocrates for 60-370 B.C. showing the close relationship between man and disease pattern in space and time.

Nutrition and human health is much more important aspect of developing countries to be solved on priority basis. It is the land which provides food to the people and its misuse will result in the shortage of food supply, which may lead to mal- and under-nutrition and related deficiency diseases. A mal- and under-nourished person may not be much productive rather than maybe liability. Therefore, nutrition deficiency leads to morbidity and poor health condition and in long term may cause death. The study of nutrition attracted Medical Geographers. Because research with regard to diet and nutrition has been done within the specific local situation. In fifties the problem of mal-nutrition and related diseases attracted many writers like Jacques May (1950). Ecology of mal-nutrition, De Castro's (1952) The geography of hunger, Learmonth's publication (1956) on nutrition levels of poor Indian diets. May and McLellan (1968) nutrition and economic development in which they point out that mal-nutrition, lower the body resistance to various diseases and, therefore, it is essential to educate people regarding the nutritive value of various local food. Whereas Davis has emphasized the need of food (1971) right food to keep fit, Swaminathan's (1975) has emphasized the need of integrated nutrients supply system. Vehassett (1983) establishes the relationship among food habits, disease and mortality in the study of health geography of France and the Benelux countries.

In India, Department of Geography, Aligarh also played its role in promoting the subject by publishing research articles on nutrition and deficiency diseases. Prof. Shafi (1967) in the field of nutrition has provided a platform to others to take the work ahead. In 1970s many contributions have been made in nutrition and deficiency diseases such as Siddique's (1971) concentration on deficiency diseases in Uttar Pradesh, Ali's contribution on the subject during (1970-80) decades, e.g. a book on food and nutrition, situation of agriculture food and nutrition in rural India, food production in India. Farooqui's Diet and Deficiency Diseases in Trans Rapti Plain, author's (1978) dietary habits in Sultanpur and the changes in production and distribution of foodgrain protein in Uttar Pradesh. Akhtar's (1981) Environment Agriculture and Nutrition in Kumoan. While in 1980s not much have been done in U.P. rather articles appear on diet and disease in context of cultural aspects (Chakravati 1982). Mishra Dube (1985) worked on nutritional level of rural settlement of Sagar District of M.P. and Pant (1992-95) studied nutritional status and deficiency diseases on Kota-dun, Uttar Pradesh, Himalaya and nutritional availability pattern of Scheduled Tribe of Buksha in Uttranchal.

The Central Ganga-Ghaghra Doab, comprising the districts of Faizabad, Ambedkar Nagar and Sultanpur lies between 26° and 26° 52′ 00″ north latitudes and 81° 32′ 00″ and 83° 10′ 00″ east longitudes. It covers an area of 8.946 sq km (Fig. 1.1). The total population of the area is 7,330,636 giving a density of 820 persons per sq km.

It appears from the available records that the area under cultivation in the Central Ganga-Ghaghra Doab accounts for about three-quarters of the total area and has encroached in some parts upon the land needed

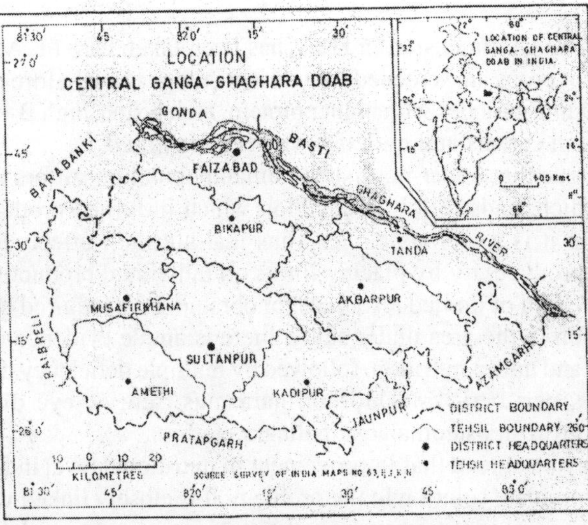

Fig. 1.1 : Location : Central Ganga-Ghaghra Doab

for fodder or pastures. The share is low where the large barren land exists as is seen in Akbarpur. As a part of the green revolution, much attention is devoted to intensive and extensive cultivation of foodgrains. While increasing the present rate of production is the immediate need of the hour, proper selection of food crops is equally important. Where one is seen on obtaining maximum benefit from any foodstuff, its nutritive value should be the chief consideration. Other considerations should be of secondary and tertiary importance. In this effort it is important that all factors which can adversely affect the total yield of food crops are to be kept under control.

There has now been intensive effort to introduce multiple cropping system, relay cropping, inter-cropping and multiple cropping systems appropriate to each region as these measures have dual advantage of improving soil fertility through introduction of leguminous crop in the cycle and also improving the nutritional level of the population through diversification of diet and increased availability of millets, pulses and oilseeds. There has been enough encouragement in increasing oilseeds through the introduction of high yielding varieties.

But side by side there has been a disturbing trend in pulses production which is the rich source of protein, particularly after the introduction of HYV of cereals, though greater areas are coming under cereals at the cost of pulse crops.

Nutritional dimension in HYV has been taken care of. All HYV varieties of crops are screened for nutrient composition before release. High yielding varieties with higher protein, high lysine, high B-crotene, high iron in cereals and millets have been identified.

It is true that under-nourished human population suffers from ill health which leads to low production which in turned produces ill-health. So it is a vicious circle. Thus mal-nutrition affects level of national productivity by placing limits on individual productivity.

As a result of limited resources for obtaining the required quantity of nutrition in the area under study, there is ample evidence of mal-nutrition and under-nutrition, followed by multiple deficiency diseases (anaemia, beri-beri, kwashiorkor/marasmus, scurvy, eye diseases, retarded growth, osteomalacia, pellagra etc.)

It may be agreed that improvement in nutritional level in the area is not a complete solution to the problem. It is closely linked with the ecological constraints as human mal-nutrition and associated diseases are ecological problems resulting in several overlapping and interacting factors in the communities. Further, mal-nutrition is closely related to the more complex problem of poverty, religion and socio-economic inequality. It cannot, therefore, be successfully solved in isolation but will have to be tackled through an integrated approach to the study of the ecological factors along with socio-economic development. Moreover, a clear understanding of the various causative or co-existing factors is also necessary.

The planning for an adequate food supply, satisfactory diet, favourble environmental conditions and the eradication of the related deficiency diseases emphasize the need for a careful detailed survey of the dietary habits and the deficiency diseases prevalent in the area.

The precise knowledge of the factors controlling or determining the existing health conditions may enable one to obtain a correct picture of the total intake of different nutrients per head per day.

Lastly, in the present work an attempt has been made by the author to study the dietary habits of the village community and the spatial distribution of nutritional deficiency diseases in the Central Ganga-Ghaghara Doab which are also related to environmental factors. Field studies relating to representative villages of the area have been undertaken by the author and the distributional pattern of the nutritional deficiency diseases has been investigated. Based upon this enquiry, relationship between the environmental factors and the spread of such disease, some valuable conclusions have been drawn.

REFERENCES

1. UNO, Department of Social Affairs, Preliminary Report on the World Social Situation with Reference to Standard of Living, New York, 1952, IV-II, p. 180.
2. The district Ambedkar Nagar has been bifurcated from Faizabad district of the Central Ganga-Ghaghara Doab.

2 Environmental Base of Agriculture and Food Production

The Central Ganga–Ghaghara Doab structurally forms part of the Indo-Gangetic Plain, varying in width from 144 km to nearly 480 km and has a length of 2400 km forming a part of north Indian peninsula. The geology of the area does not reveal anything striking except the ordinary Gengetic alluvial formation of Pleistocene to sub-recent alluvial deposits of the rivers. Beds were found of the same characteristics, alternation of sand and silt, followed by the occasional bands of Kankar and coarse send in the bottom of the bore.

On the whole, the alluvial deposits may be classified into two distinct categories. Firstly, *bhangar* or older deposits and secondly, *khadar* or the newer deposits. *Bhangar* is usually rich in concretion and covers the elevated portion of the plain (above the flood level). In general, *bhangar* lands are found at a height of 4.57 to 6.09 m above the flood level of the river. Beds of the Ghaghara and the Ganga have enough deposits of *Kankar*, derived from older rocks of different categories or from fragments of limestone contained in the alluvium[1].

Alkaline, afflorescence patches, which are due to general slope of the land and the composition of the alluvium show the general character of the *bhangar* lands. Alkaline formations are explained by the fact that the dominant constituent of the old alluvium is clay and sodium clay, reacting with the *Kankar* nodules, is turned into calcium clay, liberating sodium carbonate[2]. But the slope at several places is not more than a 30.48 cm per 1.609 km and the gradient of the water table associated with these gentle slopes is also small. These low gradients lead to a sluggish movement of the ground and surface water and results in the leaching of mineral nutrients. They are washed and deposited in deeper horizons of the soil during the monsoons, but the rate of leaching is almost stopped in summers, extensive evaporation exerts a capillary pull on the solution in the pore spaces of the soil on reaching the ground.

Khadar lands occupy a lower level in comparison to bhangar and is liable to inundation during the floods. Its level is in conformity with the principal, as the river gets older, its deposits will be younger and with the sinking of the bed, these deposits occupy a level lower than the earlier[3]. These depositions in turn lead to the depletion of soil fertility, as the Ghaghara *khadar* is less fertile than the Gomati *khadar*. *Khadar* lands are free from *Kankar* and *reh*. However, there are considerable variations in the deposits of the Ghaghara, the Ganga and the Gomati. In the deposit of the Ghaghara, which is more violent in nature, brings more sand, whereas the Ganga and the Gomati pile up mud. Floods in the Ganga are useful to the cultivators, though they often destroy the standing crops. However, they increase the fertility of the soil by adding fertile silt, but flood in the Ghaghara is undesirable and ruins the standing crops and soils both.

Drainage

The drainage of the area is closely related to its slope, except the Ghaghara, which is almost straight, rest of the rivers have tendency to follow zig-zag courses, across the plain, forming meanders and ox-bow lakes. Surface drainage is divided into two parts; first part deals with the rivers and the second with the lakes and ponds. Main rivers of the area are the Ghaghara, Gomati, Tons and Sai. Except the Ghaghara, the rest of the rivers have their origins in plains. Distribution of water in tributaries varies from nothing in hot seasons to thousands of cubic centimetres during the monsoons.

The Ghaghara is the biggest and most important river of the area, forming the northern boundary of the district Faizabad, touching the district at the village Pasia, lying in the north-west of Faizabad and leaves it at the extreme east end of Pargana Birhar. It has the tendency to change its course frequently. Right bank of the river is strong and high enough to face the danger of flood, but the left bank is pliable. Width of the river varies from 3.2 km to 4.8 km during the rains[4]. It is a perennial river as it takes its water from the Tibetan mountain.

The chief water streams, which join the Ghaghara, are Thirwa, Pikia, Saryu and Tonri, flowing the different directions and are helpful in agricultural pursuits, but off and on, they also prove to be disastrous for the standing crops in the catchment areas or near by during the period of flood of heavy rain. Their volume of water varies from little in summers to full with the onset of the monsoons.

Tons

It is the next important river of the district Faizabad. It is a perennial stream; its water decreases in summer, but during the monsoons, it attains a good size and often causes damage to life and property.

Gomati

It flows in the extreme south-west for the short distance in the district of Faizabad, but it is the main river of district Sultanpur. It joins the district Sultanpur near the village *Majhgaon*. Its channels are fairly well-marked and beds are considerably deep. Two rivers join the Gomati; one of the *Sai* on the left bank and the other is *Nand*, which joins Gomati, before it merges itself in the Ganga.

Lakes

Apart from the rivers and their tributaries, the role played by the lakes and other water bodies in the area is also considerably important. They are divided into two classes according to their origin. Firstly, those which are the outcome of meandering action of the rivers and generally work as a reservoir for the surface drainage as well as the rain water either brought by the seasonal drainage or deposited directly, emptying its excess water into the river so long as the rivers themselves do not attain flood levels. Such lakes are found in the vicinity of the rivers *Gomati*, *Bisui* and *Tonri*, whereas the second category of lakes consists of those depressions, which are isolated and collect water during the rains, e.g. *Tal Masian*, *Chitan Tal*, *Karhua Jhil*, *Raja Ka Bandh* etc.

Physical Divisions

On the basis of relief and surface drainage, the area can be divided into three physical divisions (Fig.2.1).

1. The Khadar
2. The Bhangar
3. The Region of the Lakes

1. *The Khadar* : The Khadar occupies a tract of different width and length along the rivers Ghaghara and Gomati. It is characterized by general moist conditions, so much so that in rains, it may even turn into swamps, but in winters, upper soil gets dry while the sub-soil remains moist and water can be found just by digging a few feet deep. The *Kharif* crops of these areas are subject to flood conditions, while *rabi* crops experience the deficiency of surface moisture. In short, the agriculture of the area is completely on the mercy of rains and river action. Sometimes river action captures a little portion of the fertile land by cutting channels across it, on the other hand it may deposit layers of fertile silt on what was formerly poor soil.

The Ghaghara Khadar is some what different from the Gomati Khadar. It is also known as *Manjha* and marked by large expense of waste land, covered with a thick wild growth of *Jhau* (Tamarisk) and (Thatching grass), giving shelters to wild life[5].

The Gomati Khadar is also known as *tarai*, less vulnerable to floods in comparison to the former and presents a continuous tract throughout the bank and is dissected by ravines at several places, affecting the drainage of the area especially between *Sultanpur* and *Aldeman*. *Gomati Khadar* also formed a narrow strip between upland region and lake region in the south, north and north –west, providing rich soil with restricted drainage suited to the cultivation of transplanted rice[6].

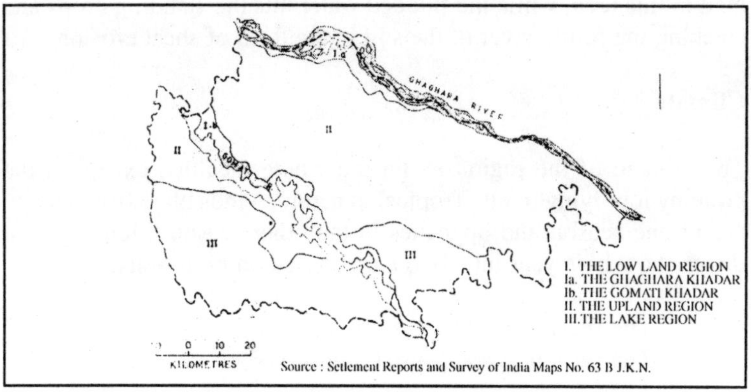

Fig. 2.1 : Location : Central Ganga-Ghaghara Doab : Physical Division

2. *The Bhangar* : It occupies the north and south-west portion of river Gomati. The portion lying north of Gomati contains three main types of soil, viz., sandy, loam and clayey loam, but these concentrations are rather in patches, and it is difficult to mark them on the map. Sandy soil is generally found in the south–west of Gomati as well as on the right bank of the Ghaghara. Its width varies from 1.5 to 5 km[7], but the predominant soil is sandy-loam, containing enough moisture. The chief crop of this area is *arhar*, but is vulnerable to frost. The central part between sandy soil area to the north and south of this area is covered with loam, good for agricultural practices, coupled with easy irrigation facilities. Clayey-loam is found near the lake region in the south-east corner and also in the central part in patches, containing lakes and depressions. Between *Gomati Khadar* and south Lake region exists the narrow strip with fertile soil, devoted to transplanted rice, traversed by numerous small streams, which join Gomati. Water table of this area is said to be at a depth of 6 to 8 m but in the monsoon season it comes a little up.

3. *The Region of Lakes:* It covers the south and south-west along with the south-eastern corner of Sultanpur district (Fig.2.1). South and south-west portion is agriculturally poor owing to barren lands and *swamps*, coupled with numerous lakes and ponds. Only rice can be cultivated on profitable basis. The south-eastern portion is covered by clayey soil, but it has also patches of barren land and alike southern portion, here too barren lands exist. Due to the presence of *reh*, even the cultivated patches give poor results. Water-logging, due to bad drainage in the rainy season, leads to the formation of barren (*usar*) land in this area, while the flooded water hits the standing crops and leaching the fertile layer of the soil in the form of sheet erosion.

Climate

The climate of the region is, on the whole, healthy, except in the swampy low-lying tracts. Tropical in nature, winds blow from land to sea in one season and opposites in the other season. Meteorologist divide the whole year into Two Parts, based on monsoons.

(a) The season of north-east monsoons.
(b) The season of south-west monsoons[8].

(a) The season of north-east monsoon is further sub-divided into two parts: (i) cold weather season lasting from January to February (ii) hot weather season, begins with March and lasts till mid-June.

(b) The season of south-west monsoon is also sub-divided into two parts: (i) the season of general rains, from mid-June to October. (ii) The season of retreating monsoon, commencing from November to December. Cold season refers to the period of *rabi* crops, whereas *kharif* crops coincide with the rainy season.

Broadly speaking, the climate of the area is divided into three distinct seasons.

(1) The cold weather season (November to February),
(2) The hot weather season (March to mid-June), and
(3) The season of rains (mid-June to October).

The Cold Weather Season

During the early November, almost half of the high pressure belt moves from north-western India, covering the whole Ganga-Ghaghara Doab. The direction of the winds from west to east is the result of pressure distribution in general and partly influenced by the Himalayan relief[9]. The mean monthly temperature in the month of December at Faizabad was 15.6°C whereas at Sultanpur, it was recorded as 16.4°C, but the lowest temperature of the year was recorded 3.4°C, whereas the highest temperature touched 46.0°C in the Central Ganga-Ghaghara Doab[10]. The days are fairly warm, while the nights are cold. January is considered to be the coldest month of the year, accompanied by *mist* and *fog,* known as '*kohra*'; often reduces the visibility to almost nil. Frost is also noticed frequently, but its intensity varies. Often crops are affected. February is the month of clear sky with increasing temperature, but still remains colder than November. During the span of December to February, thunder storms move through this area and early light rain in this season is expected which is a boon to the crops, but rains accompanied by hailstorms are fatal to the standing crops. Relative humidity varies between 64 per cent and 69 per cent at Faizabad while 52 per cent and 53 per cent at Sultanpur.[11]

The Hot Weather Season

Months of March, April, May and half of June, constitute rest half of the dry monsoon. Sharp rise in temperature occurs in March; in this month, the mean monthly temperature rises to 24.0°C, while the mean maximum temperature remains 32.0°C, and the mean minimum temperature 15.0° (Fig. 2.2). Increase in temperature continues up to the month of May. The thermometer registers a high temperature and the mean monthly temperature in May at Faizabad and Sultanpur remains 31.9°C and 33.8°C respectively, but the relative humidity drops to 29 per cent and 23 per cent at Faizabad and Sultanpur respectively.[12] The days are hot, while the nights are warm, though the mean diurnal range of temperature is as high as in March.

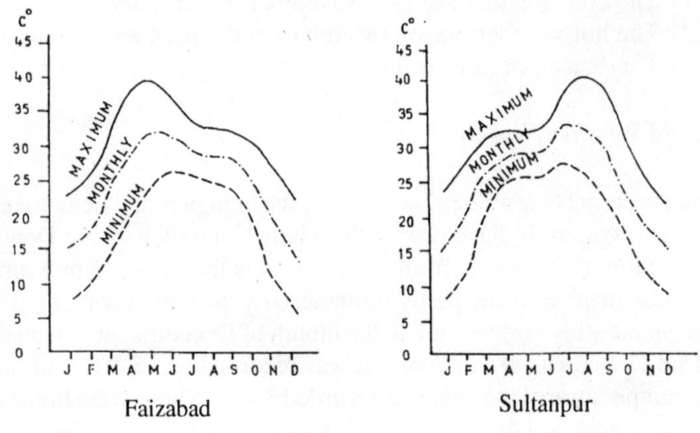

Source : Climatological Tables, Indian Meteorological Department, 2001

Fig. 2.2 : Mean Monthly Temperatures

May experience the highest temperature of the year. The mean maximum temperature during this month are 31.4°C and 34.1°C respectively, while an absolute maximum of 40°C is not uncommon.[13] The excessive heat has a desiccating influence on the vegetation, and the surface becomes parched. May and half of June is the period of intense hot dry westerly winds, locally known as *loo*. Sometimes it becomes so vigorous that humidity comes down to two or three per cent between 12 noon and 4:00 p.m.[14]

Due to strong local disturbances, some sporadic, short lived rain can be seen; it may be repeated frequently also. The barometric oscillations during a storm are rapid and considerable, but are largely due to local courses.[15]

The total average rainfall in hot weather season varies between 35.8 mm and 34.3 mm, but the number of days and the amount of rainfall is higher in May with 51.8 to 42.7 mm, whereas the lowest recorded rainfall in April in case of Faizabad is 24.7 mm and 26.4 mm in case of Sultanpur during March.[16] These rains are good for the maize and fodder crops of the area. It has the tendency to decrease from east to west, due to the increasing sea distance as the air gets drier and gradually easterlies are replaced by the westerlies, reducing the precipitation accompanied by the storms. Rainfall received during hot weather season gives temporary relief from heat as well as helps in sowing of early rice crop. However, rains with violent winds cause damage to the trees, buildings etc.

The Season of General Rains

The climate of the area closely resembles that of the rest of Ganga-Ghaghara Doab and calls for no special comment. The wet monsoons normally start from the middle of June and last till October. The rainfall in the area is distinctly heavy, when compared with the other districts, but the average is not higher than that recorded in the trans-Ghaghara districts to the north, which lie closer to the hills. With the arrival of monsoon in the area, a drastic change in temperature and humidity conditions is noticed. Rainfall alternating with rainless gaps of a day or two is common in the months of July and August and these are the rainiest months of the year as they receive more than 50 per cent of the total annual rainfall. The month of September is the period of long rainless gaps with the slight rise in day temperature. Humidity, however, remains high with no motion in air. The average rainfall of these three districts, viz., Faizabad, Ambedkar Nagar and Sultanpur in this month is recorded as 196.7 mm,198.5 mm and 184.9 mm (Fig. 2.3) respectively, while in June alone all the districts received 106.5 mm, 108.7 mm and 82.2 mm respectively. High humidity with close weather conditions makes the heat intolerable and creates a number of problems for health. The time between September to half of October is considered to be the most unhealthy period of the year. October is the month of retreating monsoon, but the mean maximum temperature remains as high as in September. Rainfall, though little, is useful for the *rabi* crops and for the maturity of late rice. Rainfall in the months of June and September is irregular, affecting the agricultural practices of *kharif* and *rabi* seasons, whereas continuous rainfall for several days leads to flood conditions, resulting in sheet and gully erosion, and destruction of crop and dwellings.

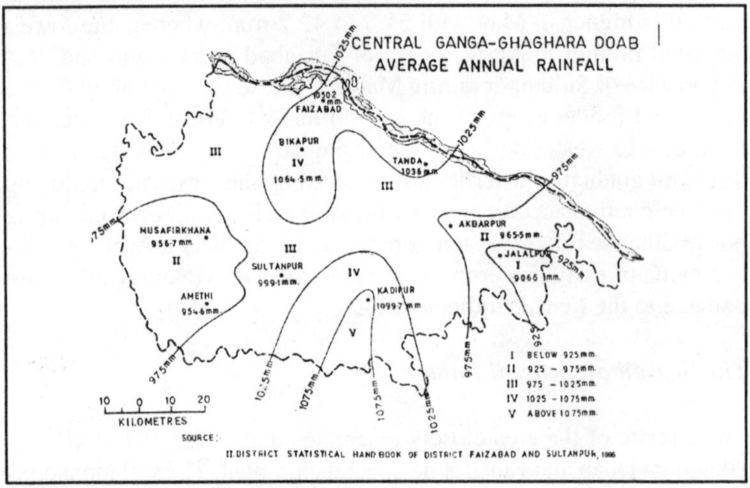

Fig. 2.3 : Average Annual Rainfall

Annual Variability

Annual variability means the percentages of mean variations from the average, half the difference of the two means; firstly, for the years of excess rainfall to the average, secondly, for the years it has short of the average rainfall, calculated by the author with the help of rainfall data for 50 years 1951–2000.

$$\frac{UQ - LQ}{M \times 2}$$

Where,

UQ = Upper quartile
LQ = Lower quartile
M = Median

It can be seen from the mean annual variability of rainfall is greatest in the north-western part of the area, i.e. from Tanda towards Bikapur and is lowest in the east. It is noticed that variability is high, where the rainfall is low and with high rainfall, variability is low of course with some exceptions. Twenty two per cent variability is noticed at Musafir Khana, where the rainfall is 956.7 mm. Whereas 17 per cent is reported at Khadipur with the rainfall of 1086.7 mm. It is good that variability at no station is recorded below 17 per cent as 12 per cent or below, variability is said to be susceptible to famine. The driest years known were 1876 and 1877 with 530.35 and 519.43 mm of rainfall respectively, a deficiency which resulted in famine of some intensity.[17]

Variability in the Wet Monsoon (*June to October*)

Agriculture activities are much dependent on variability in the wet monsoon than annual variability. Timely distribution of rainfall is more important, even if the average rainfall is below the normal. If the rainfall is in time, the crops will not be much affected. Such as heavy or scarcity of rainfall in June affects the sowing of the early *kharif* crops and also their output. Sufficient amount of rainfall in July and August is harmful for rice crop. Deficiency in rainfall in the months of September and October delays sowing of winter crops and adversely affects the yield and quality of the late *kharif* crops. Heavy rainfall during these months leads to water logging, while premature cessation of the rains may cause postponement or restriction to the sowing of the *rabi* crops.

Table 2.1 : Showing the percentage Mean Monthly Variability at Selected Stations*

Station	*June*	*July*	*August*	*September*	*October*
Faizabad	59	31	24	49	351
Akbarpur	47	35	30	38	255
Bikapur	35	27	23	40	312
Tanda	55	29	26	36	213
Jalalpur	53	26	32	50	132
Sultanpur	55	30	21	46	313
Amethi	80	35	25	46	146
Kadipur	40	37	27	38	184
Musafir Khan	54	28	27	45	111

* Calculated on the basis of monthly rainfall stations of 50 years (1951-2000) for the selected stations. Published by Govt. of India. Monthly and Annual Rainfall Table of Uttar Pradesh, Lucknow.

It is clear from Table 2.1 that the variability is least in the months of July and August, but is higher in the rest of three months. In the months of July and August, variability is below 35 per cent, with exception at Kadipur (37 per cent) and the lowest is reported at Sultanpur with 21 per cent. In June, variability fluctuates between 40 and 59 per cent; with the exceptions at Bikapur, where it is 35 per cent while at Amethi it is 80 per cent. The month of October experience very high range of variability, i.e. (111-351), whereas in September and June it range between 38-80 per cent (except at Bikapur and Tanda 35 and 36 per cent respectively).

The present study has shown that rainfall is more variable in October and less variable in the months of September and June. Variability is high at the time when its regularity is most required in the Central Ganga-Ghaghara *Doab*. Such conditions may lead to uncertainties in the agricultural programme.

Soils

Data based on scientific classification of soils are not available. However, we have some information about the soils of the area which is based on the settlement reports and the District Gazetteers. The main considerations in such classification where texture, colour, availability of water and the level of land.[18] Local names were given to each type of soil and are still accepted in the Central Ganga-Ghaghara Doab.

On the basis of mechanical classification of soils, introduced in 1860, soils are classified as *loam* (*doras* or *dumat* locally known) *clay* (*matiyar*) and *sand* (*bhur*). Later on, this system was changed and a new mode of classification based on productivity and fertility was adopted according to which the soils of the area are grouped into three categories: (i) Goind, (ii) Miyana and (iii) Palo.

Geologically, the soils of Central Ganga-Ghaghara Doab fall in two parts: (i) *Khadar* or new alluvium and (ii) *Bhangar* or old alluvium.

(i) The Khadar lands : They are found on either side of the Ghaghara and Gomati banks, and their texture varies from clay to sand or silty sand. River in spate carries large quantities of materials of all sizes from coarse sand to fine silt and with the retarded speed coarser sand is deposited.[19] As the distance increase from the banks, texture improves with greater percentage of clay and silt.

(ii) Bhangar lands : They are found along the high bank of the river Ghaghara in the north and its belt varies from about 2 km to 5 km in width.[20] Such lands are generally free from

floods as they occupy the higher parts of the area. Five varieties of soils are found in the entire *bhangar* lands. They are (i) Sandy soils, (ii) Sandy loam, (iii) Loam, (iv) Clayey loam and (v) Clay. Such soils are evenly distributed in the *bhangar* lands of the area (Fig. 2.4).

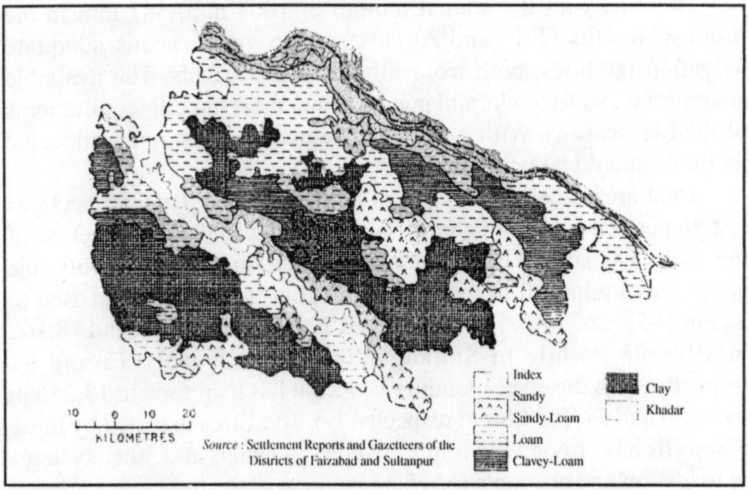

Fig. 2.4 : Soils

Usar Soils : The term *usar* is also in common use, applied to the barren lands infected with saline efflorescence known as *reh*. It has a very irregular distribution in the Central Ganga-Ghaghara Doab and is not possible to mark their exact areas on soil map. However, their good portion is found in the south, east and south-west areas of the district Sultanpur, whereas in Faizabad district, it is confined to a few patches. Its formation is due to the presence of the efflorescence of Sodium Carbonate and Sulphate, found in abundance in the alluvial soils of the Indo-Gangetic plain.[21]

Irrigation

Irrigation plays an important role in the promotion of agriculture. It is one of the many measures to increase output and to make full use of the land by growing second and third crop in the same field. It is extremely essential for cash crops and vegetable. Naturally, in the absence of good irrigation, one has to depend upon the nature and the amount of rainfall which often falls short of the requirement coupled with unevenly distribution and irregularities which compels the farmers to produce merely single crop. Most of the agricultural lands of the area receive fair supply of irrigation water, but security and timely supply depends rather on the nature of the sources from which water is obtained.

The area with the annual rainfall of 1004 mm, 587 mm in the rainiest months (July and August) of the year[22] needs adequate irrigation facilities, both from tubewells and canals. The available sources, i.e., wells, tanks and ponds cannot meet the full requirements of the two seasons. With a view to safeguard against risks, adequate facilities should be provided.

Total area covered by various canals is about 161,256 hectares (32.86 per cent), i.e. Ghaghara, Sarda, Tanda canals. Construction of tubewells has started in recent years. Till 1946, there was only one government tubewell in the whole area, but its number increased to 245 in 1958, 267 in 1963, and touched 22,930 in 1984-85, and 78,192 in 1994-95,[23] while in Sultanpur the numbers were 75 and 91 respectively in the corresponding years but has increased to 13,266 in 1984-85 and 58,428 (94-95 respectively). Total area irrigated by these tubewells has crossed the limits covered by canals and other systems of irrigation and accounts for 75.83 per cent of the total irrigated area of 675,933 hectares in the districts. Construction of private tubewells has also increased tremendously to 314,767 in Faizabad, followed by Sultanpur district with 150,857 by the year 1994-95. Construction of wells has almost stopped and its utility has also decreased. Tanks and ponds still continue to be some source of water supply but their use in agriculture has been reduced with the introduction of more and more tubewells and expansion of canal system. Moreover tanks and ponds are rapidly waning away.

Agriculture

Agriculture being the most important occupation in Uttar Pradesh, a large percentage of the population of this area (approximately 80 per cent) depends on it. There is a rapid increase in the growth rate of population not only in the area under study, but in the entire country whereas the rate of productivity is relatively low with the result that adequate food supplies cannot be ensured for the entire population. Moreover, on account of unstable economy, people cannot afford to eat such foods which can supply them with essential nutrients. So that they may not fall easy victim to various deficiency diseases. The author is of opinion that the present situation can be improved to an appreciable extent with the application of modern techniques based on a scientific survey of agricultural lands and suitability of crops to different types of soils.

Agriculture in the Central Ganga-Ghaghara Doab attains a satisfactory position in comparison to other districts of eastern Uttar Pradesh. The area is endowed with very good soils, suitable climate for a variety of agricultural productions and some irrigation water. Despite these facts, the cropping intensity is low and the population of the area finds it difficult to get proper and adequate food supplies. Recent trends have shown that continuous efforts are being made to put more and more lands under cultivation and to produce variety of crops with increased output with the help of modern techniques, seeds, fertilizers etc.

The system of agriculture in no way differs from that in the surrounding districts and the crops are sown in the customary rotation; the produce is more or less the same in value as that obtained in similar lands elsewhere. With the abolition of bonded labour, introduction of consolidation scheme and ceilings on land holdings, the interest in agriculture has increased as it makes way for better planning by using tractors, tube-wells and other techniques.

The different geographical environments prevailing in different regions makes it almost impossible to find out any agreed solution to anyone problem on State level. Each region has its own individuality and therefore, needs separate treatment. Regional diversities affect the agricultural land use too[24]. With a view to assess the agricultural potentialities of the region, it is essential to embark on a plan which takes into account soil, climate and socio-economic factors of the area. Table 2.2 gives a detailed picture of land utilization in the area. About 65.7 per cent, i.e. 579,829 hèctares of the total reported area is actually sown in 1994-95 which is short by 3.33 per cent in comparison to 1974-75, 69.03 per cent, i.e. 609,651 hectares. This is also obvious from this table that total actually sown area of Faizabad (68.4 per cent) was relatively less than that of Sultanpur (69.3 per cent) in 1973-74. However in 1994-85, the reported area of Faizabad increased from 437,760 to 442,694, +0.13 per cent while the sown area decreased from 68.4 per cent to 67.05 per cent. Comparing the figures for the two districts, it is obvious that despite decrease in the sown area in the case of Faizabad, the percentage is still higher than that of Sultanpur.

Table 2.2 : Land Utilization in the Central Ganga-Ghaghara Doab in the year 1973-74 and 1994-95[25]

District	*Year*	*Utilised Land*	*Forest*	*Usar*	*Land in other Uses*	*Cultivable Waste*	*Pastures*	*Groves*	*Fallow Land*	*Other Fallow Land*	*Actual Sown Area*
Faizabad	1973-74	437,760	1,394	10,643	50,235	23,520	495	27,252	15,483	9,383	299,355
	1994-95	442,694	1,234	7,530	62,349	9,330	2208	17,331	28,119	17,759	296,834
Sultanpur	1973-74	445,370	1,643	27,348	40,209	20,601	517	19,702	13,932	11,122	310,296
	1994-95	440,180	1,789	15,478	50,088	13,208	2,399	7,868	41,578	24,777	282,995
Total	1973-74	883,130	3,037	37,991	90,444	40,121	1,012	46,954	29,415	20,505	609,651
	1994-95	882,874	3,023	23,008	112,437	22,538	4,607	25,199	79,697	42,536	579,829

However, with reclamation of *usar* lands and using the cultivable waste land including fallow land, more areas can be added to the existing cultivated land. Thus more food can be made available to the local population of this area.

The main purpose of soil classification is to determine the nature of crops to be grown in the area under study. Cropping patterns that have evolved under the present soil condition reflect a close relationship between the physical environment and the socio-economic conditions. The existing cropping pattern reveals that sugarcane is the most important cash crop, while rice, wheat, barley, gram, peas etc. are other important crops. The main *rabi* crops are wheat, barley, peas, gram and pulses. Among *kharif* crops rice is the leading crop followed by millets and maize.

Table 2.3 shows that the most important of all *kharif* crops is rice, which covers major portion of the net sown area of 347,809 hectares (1994-95), which is +81,421 hectares (30 per cent) more than the area reported during 1973-74. Major increase was reported during 1984-85 to 1994-95 which is 25 per cent. The increase in rice cultivation is appreciably high in Faizabad (66.6 to 83.64 per cent). In case of Sultanpur, the position is just the reverse. Cultivation of rice decreased from 126,185 (1973-74) to 103,308 hectares (-18.2 per cent) in 1984-85. But picked up again during 1984-85 to1994-95 and accounted for 53.6 per cent. Briefly speaking, the area devoted to rice in Faizabad (83.64 per cent) is more higher than the area under rice in Sultanpur (79.7 per cent). Production also has increased from 105,414 metric tonnes to 263,534 and to 407,080 so is the yield in Faizabad district, whereas in Sultanpur district increase was merely to the tune of 7,562 metric tonnes in 1984-85 but by 1994-95 it increased to 165,200 metric tonnes mainly because of tremendous increase in area . The main reason for this difference is due to better soil and drainage. The average yield of rice is more than 50 per cent higher in Faizabad than in Sultanpur (21.53 and 16.46 quintal per hectare). The survey conducted by the author indicates that the bulk of population eat rice and the coarse grain produced in the two agricultural seasons.

Wheat is the main *rabi* crop, which constitutes the main diet of well-off inhabitants, followed by other crops, e.g. gram, barley, peas, in both the districts. Wheat is sown alone as well as in combination with other crops, e.g. barley and gram, but the most popular combination is with barley. Wheat alone accounts for 87.91 and 81.97 per cent of the cultivated land in the *rabi* season during the year

Table 2.3 : Production and Yield of Crops in the Kharif Season in 1973-74, 1984-85 and 1994-95[26]
Area in hectares, Production in metric tones, Yield in quintals per hectare

		Faizabad			*Sultanpur*		
Crops	*Year*	*Area*	*Production*	*Yield*	*Area*	*Production*	*Yield*
Rice	1973-74	140,203	105,414	7.43	126,185	88,511	7.07
(347,809)	1984-85	174,831	263,534	15.07	103,308	96,073	9.30
	1994-95	189,112	407,080	21.53	158,697	261,273	16.46
Jowar Bajra	1973-74	9,180	6,332	7.02	40,565	11,091	7.02
	1984-85	8,674	9,921	13.74	30,140	42,286	14.80
	1994-95	5,187	3,722	98.95	10,586	9,661	10.02
Maize	1973-74	9,932	2,922	2.94	6,388	1,880	2.94
	1984-85	4,312	2,965	6.08	2,918	1,649	5.65
	1994-95	2,605	3,774	14.49	5,227	7.574	14.49
Sawan, Kondon	1973-74	13,932	7,429	5.26	11.045	5,425	5.26
	1984-85	1,977	891	4.86	3,699	2,635	6.76
	1994-95	33	24	7.41	337	250	7.41
Arhar (Pegion	1973-74	5,787	7,270	12.56	14,695	3,348	20.65
Pea)	1984-85	9,563	9,046	9.46	12,425	26,751	21.53
	1994-95	8,478	8,629	10.18	11,235	9,299	8.28
Pulses (Urd,	1973-74	1,352	384	—	5,852	1,633	—
Moong, Moth)	1984-85	1,002	218	2.66	3,335	820	2.66
	1994-95	440	169	—	2,948	1,130	—
Sugarcane	1973-74	21,913	629,216	287.14	9,713	303,529	312.50
	1984-85	20,436	840,083	411.08	7,791	297,554	381.82
	1994-95	20,235	1,001,794	495.08	10,008	528,342	527.92

1994-95 with an average yield of 25.30 and 22.03 tonnes in the districts of Faizabad and Sultanpur respectively (Table 2.4). In Faizabad, the area under wheat has increased to 125 per cent in the last twenty years whereas in Sultanpur, it is up by 183 per cent and increased in production by 422.5 per cent (67,419 to 352,284 metric tonnes) whereas Faizabad with only about 125 per cent increase of land has produced more than 371 per cent of wheat (98,164 to 462,148 metric tonnes) followed by gram, peas and potato, the other important crops of the *rabi* season.

Population

According to the 2001 census, the total population of the two districts, viz., Faizabad (including Ambedkar Nagar) and Sultanpur was 7,304,213.[27] Further, about 89 per cent and 96 per cent respectively of the total population lived in the villages. There has been slight decrease in the rural population. It has decreased to the tune of 4.5 and 3.2 per cent in the districts of Faizabad and Sultanpur from 1971 to 2001. But the overall increase in population is positive as it is evident from Table 2.5.

Table 2.5 shows that after 1901 onward till 2001, there has been regular increase in the population of this area, except in the year 1911 and 1921 when the area witnessed emigration from here to Burma, West Indies, Fiji Islands, Malaysia, Singapore etc. in search of employment and also a large number of people died of epidemic diseases during the said period.

The entire population of the area is divided into cultivators, agricultural labourers and people engaged in house-hold industries and other activities, of which 63.15 per cent are cultivators followed by 20.8 per cent agricultural labourers. Only 3.76 per cent of the population is engaged in house-hold industries and the rest is engaged in non-agricultural activities. What is striking a noteworthy is that an appreciable percentage (38.2) of the female population participates in agricultural pursuits. Percentage of workers engaged in agriculture is higher in Sultanpur (85.7 per cent) than in Faizabad (80.2 per cent). Despite all the efforts made to step up agricultural productivity under the existing environmental conditions, food problems have been solved to a limited extent. However the solution does not lie only in meeting the total food requirement of the population in the area but to ensure nutritive diets as well for them.

Table 2.4 : Production and Yield of Crops in the Rabi Season in 1973-74, 1984-85 and 1994–95[28]

		Faizabad			*Sultanpur*		
Crops	*Year*	*Area*	*Production*	*Yield*	*Area*	*Production*	*Yield*
Wheat	1973-74	81,116	98,164	12.10	56,447	67,419	11.94
	1984-85	169,885	358,153	21.08	127,257	229,601	18.04
	1994-95	182,687	462,148	25.30	159,895	352,284	22.03
Barley	1973-74	12,814	11,907	9.29	36,066	36,776	10.20
	1984-85	3,497	3,924	11.22	10,492	14,085	13.42
	1994-95	1,147	1,669	14.55	2964	4,314	14.55
Gram	1973-74	28,575	12,642	4.36	39,958	22,974	5.75
	1984-85	20,248	21,535	10.64	27,907	29.661	10.63
	1994-95	8,998	7,138	7.93	12,798	101,53	7.93
Peas	1973-74	25,139	11,252	4.48	23,049	11,085	4.81
	1984-85	7,577	6,124	8.08	8,228	5,823	7.08
	1994-95	8,670	8,687	10.02	9,617	8,396	8.73
Masur	1973-74	348	144	4.14	1,204	499	4.14
	1984-85	556	361	6.49	1,938	1,258	6.49
	1994-95	777	640	8.24	3,240	2,669	8.24
Potatoes	1973-74	4,743	44,436	93.69	4,532	42,459	93.69
	1984-85	8,248	125,089	151.66	5,287	84,486	159.80
	1994-95	5530	108938	196.99	6535	137856	210.95

Table 2.5 : Distribution of Population, its Growth (Percentage) during the period of 1901-2001[28]

	Faizabad + Ambedkar Nagar		*Sultanpur*	
Year	*Population*	*Growth*	*Population*	*Growth*
1901	1,221,894	—	1,092,273	—
1911	1,150,843	–5.81	1,056,550	–3.27
1921	1,168,617	+ 1.05	1,012,050	–4.21
1931	1,201,384	+ 2.80	1,060,055	+ 4.74
1941	1,315,728	+ 9.52	1,110,433	+ 4.75
1951	1,477,662	+12.31	1,292,949	+ 16.44
1961	1,633,359	+ 10.50	1,412,984	+ 9.28
1971	1,925, 998	+ 17.82	1,641,900	+16.20
1981	2,382,515	+ 23.70	2,042,778	+ 24.41
1991	2,978,484	+ 25.01	2,558,970	+ 25.27
2001	4,113,287	+ 27.60	3,190,926	+ 24.70

REFERENCES

1. Medlicott, H.B. and Blandford, W.T., '*A Manual of the Geology of India*', London, 1879, p. 393.
2. Auden, J.B. and Roy, P.C., '*Report on Sodium Salts in Reh Soil in Uttar Pradesh*', Records of the Geological Survey of India, Professional Paper No. 1, Calcutta 1942, p. 3.
3. Wadia, D.N., '*Geology of India*', London, 1953, p. 391.
4. Final Settlement Report of the District Faizabad, Allahabad, 1942, p. 2.
5. Final Settlement Report, *op. cit.*, p. 4.
6. District Gazetteer of Sultanpur, Allahabad, 1903, p. 15.
7. Final Settlement Report ...., *op. cit.,* 1942, p. 5.
8. Kendrew, W.G., '*The Climate of the continents*', Great Britain, 1961, p. 155.
9. Shafi, M., '*Land Utilization in Eastern Uttar Pradesh*', Aligarh, 1960, p. 16.
10. *The Climatological Tables*, Indian Meteorological Department, New Delhi, 1981.
11. *Ibid.*
12. *Ibid.*
13. Siddiqui, N.A., *Land Utilization in Central Ganga-Ghaghara Doab*, Unpublished Thesis of Ph.D, Aligarh, 1965, p. 31.
14. Blandford, H.F., '*The Climate and Weather of India*', Memoirs of the Indian Meteorological Department, Vol. VI, No. 6, 1896, pp. 162-63.
15. Blandford, H.F., *ibid.*, Vol. III, 1886-88, pp. 162-63.
16. *Memoirs of the Indian Meteorological Department*, Vol. XXXI, Part III, Simla, 1962, pp. 107.
17. Faizabad, *op. cit.*, p. 16.
18. Raychodhary, S.P. and Mukerjee, S.K., 'Present Position of Soil Survey in India', *Journal of Scientific and Industrial Research*, Vol. VI, 10, Calcutta, 1947, pp. 406.

19. Hall, A.D., Revised by Robinson, G.W., '*The Soil*', (An Introduction to the Scientific Study of the Growth of Crops) London, 1956, p. 39.
20. Final Settlement Report ......, *op. cit.*, p. 4.
21. Auden, J.B., Gupta, B.C., Ray, P.C. and Husain, M., Report on Sodium Salts in Reh Soils in United Provinces (Uttar Pradesh), Recor*ds of the Geological Survey of Ind*ia, Vol. LXXVII, No. 1, Calcutta, 1942, p. 3.
22. *Memoirs of the Indian Meteorological Department*, op. cit., pp. 65-66.
23. *Agriculture Statistics of Uttar Pradesh*, Lucknow, 1994-95 pp. 20-21
24. Ahmad, S.W., *Distribution of Nutritional Deficiency Diseases in Relation to Envlronmental Factors in Central Ganga-Ghaghara Doab*, Dissertation submitted for M. Phil Degree, Aligarh, 1975, p. 15.
25. *Source : Agricultural Bulletins of Uttar Pradesh* 1997.
26. *Ibid.*, pp. 31, 34, 38, 42, 46, 87.
27. *Ibid.*, pp. 51, 55, 59
28. Since, Final population totals, *Cencus of India*, Uttar Pradesh, 2001 Survey, 10.
28. *Census of India* 2001, Series 10, New Delhi.
29. *Census of India* 2001, Series 10, New Delhi.

3 Food Deficiency and Diseases

The science of nutrition is a very defused subject, since it cuts across a number of disciplines. The scope of nutrition is so great that it is impossible for an individual to encompass the entire field[1] . But in the study of human nutrition, geography is as important as any other natural science. It is evident that we need to know what sort of vitamins, minerals our body needs and what happens if we do not get upto the standard requirement of any one of them. It is equally necessary that we should know something about economic and geography of food production, its distribution and attitude of a group or of an individual towards food. People need to know, because nutritional health is fundamental to normal general health and the prevention or reduction in the severity of diseases. The need to know has steadily increased over the past decade due to tremendous changes in the nature of food supply and in the eating habits of the rural population of India. There need not be any inherent undesirable nutritional status of the local population in the first place and of the impact of their changing habits and lifestyle on the nutritional health. Once nutritional status determined, the information can be used as a starting point and scientific base of efforts to encourage and suggest people to improve their nutritional status wherever needed, and to continuously monitor for changes in the future.

The researcher is, firstly, interested to determine the prevalence of nutritional deficiency in any particular area on the basis of geographical location, type of community, season, agricultural practices, income level and secondly, has to highlight the underlying factors determining the food choices and degrees of variations in such patterns to re-evaluate food, which has its direct effect on health.

Nutrition and diet are not synonymous though they are popularly used in that fashion. Diet consists of various items of food which are ingested and converted for use in the body for building up and maintaining it in a vital condition. Nutrition is the end of the process by which these are assimilated and produce the desired result[2]. While nutrition is a science that deals with all the various constituents of which food is composed and the way in which proper nourishment is brought about[3]. The modern public health movement is neither concerned with the prevention of diseases nor with nutrition. It has the broader aim at creating an environment in which each individual can develop his potentialities to its full. This is particularly true as regards nutrition. Mal-nutrition produces state of ill-health and lowers the resistance and physical efficiency, Which are perhaps more important than the disease itself. Numerous investigations among school children in India have shown that a large percentage of children are in poor state of health. Again in the adult population, the ill-effects of mal-nutrition are widely evident in the shape of a low general health and reduced capacity for work.[4] The problem of proper nourishment is assuming importance day by day as recently the United Nations' (FAO) survey has revealed that the number of mal-nourshed people in the world has risen from about 455 million in 1974 to nearly 517 million in 1989 and till the end of this century it has crossed more than 1.0 billion. Preschool children, younger women and school age children suffer most often from poor nutrition, and it has accounted for 25 to 50 per cent in developing countries. The survey has found wide disparities, not only between rich and poor nations like India but also between and within individual developing countries, largely due to distribution of available food.[5]

Therefore, a positive aspect of the campaign for improved nutrition must be strongly emphasized. Freedom from disease is one thing; abundant health is another. The goal to be aimed at is the creation of a healthy and vigorous population.[6]

People often ask do potatoes make people fat or does spinach supply human beings with iron? Fish is primarily a brain food, or an apple a day keeps the doctor away; even the apple growers get sick and call the physician. It may, therefore, be concluded that none of the basic nutrients, e.g. carbohydrates, fat, protein, vitamins or minerals can alone promote a healthy growth, but a proper combination of all these nutrients is essential. It is a well known fact that the average Indian diet consists of cereals and pulses which together account for nearly three-fourths of the caloric intake. In the case of a large number of people with lower incomes, this proportion goes up. Cereals and pulses are so important in our diet that supply roughly 86 per cent of protein, most of thiamine, niacin and major portion of iron content.

Besides one-fourth of fat, their of calcium and riboflavin and some proportion of vitamin-A, C and D, rest is to be derived from other sources. However, other sources contribute almost negligible amount, e.g. fruits, green vegetables, milk and animal products. How much of each of the nutrients is required or an individual has been recommended by the nutritional experts on the basis of ethnic, climatic and socio-economic consideration as well as the type of activity, e.g. sedentary, moderate and hard worker. The suggested meal based on such considerations is known as 'balanced diet'; whenever there is any deviation from the suggested daily diet for the population, undesirable result is bound to occur.

This may be in the form of mal-nutrition or under-nutrition. Balanced diet may ensure healthy growth of men and women. A balanced diet is defined as one which contains correct proportion of all the nutrients needed by the individual. A person is said to suffer from mal-nutrition when the daily diet does not contain essential nutrients in the proportion suggested by the experts of nutritional sciences. Mal-nutrition is one of the most important health problems of the world in general and of India in particular. It is estimated that between one-half and two-third of the world's population suffer from it.[7] This is the result of either chronic insufficiency of food or of inadequacy of the protective foods necessary for a healthy life, or a combination of both situation. It may result in serious disorder like anaemia in women and blindness among the children. This general hunger or hunger for specific nutrients does a lot of damage, the effects of which are far reaching. Infants born of mal-nourished mother starts life with a handicap. In the first of two years, many of them of mal-nutrition alone or due to their state of mal-nourishment, succumb easily to gastro-intestinal and respiratory infections. The prevalence of various communicable diseases in the area which is confronted with the spectre of hunger makes the situation still more serious, for resistance to infections among the population of the area is low.

Considering the causes of mal-nutrition, it may be said that the main reasons are the prevailing poverty among the down-trodden societies and short supply of foods. But there are some more reasons also which play equally important role, i.e. ignorance, traditional foods, lack of knowledge regarding proper foods and its effect on health. According to Maxim, Dixit and Mudambi (1969), health depends upon (i) adequate food, (ii) quality of food, (iii) appropriate balance in regard to essential food constituents."[8]

According to May (1961), most of the patients are from the poor classes of people living on diets that are both qualitatively and quantitatively inadequate.[9] Corwin (1949) accepted the diets of the villagers adequate for the most part, but an adequate diet does not, of course, ensure adequate nutrition,[10] and the diets of poor nutritional quality are directly responsible for the occurrence of specific diseases.[11]

Non-Nutrition Causes of Mal-Nutrition

Though diet plays an important role, even then when diet is proper from nutritional viewpoint, mal-nutrition may occur due to non-nutritional causes, because the causes of mal-nutrition are always complex. It is important to realise this complex position, for the same type of mal-nutrition may be caused by different factors and it is essential to find out such factors to plan a preventive programme relevant to local conditions. In recent years, the role of infections and infestations in the causation of mal-nutrition coupled with helping environmental conditions have been well documented. Indian villages are among the main suffers due to their gloomy physical conditions. Certain state of mal-nutrition develops, which does not show sign until developed fully. Many infections occur more easily, persist longer and cause much higher mortality in mal-nourished children.

Infectious diseases play an important role in the initiation of mal-nutrition itself. Deep-rooted cultural beliefs, customs and dependence on out-dated and tradition bound methods of treatment play a definite part in the causation of mal-nutrition.[12] The crude and unscientific methods may not only harmful in themselves but also pose great danger by preventing people to seek immediate medical attention by qualified personnel.

Mal-Nutrition

Single deficiency almost apparently never occurs in human beings because even simply unrefined foods, e.g. milk might supply forty nutrients, may be roughly enough. A person whose diet is faulty suffers from multiple and overlapping deficiencies simultaneously. A single deficiency can, however, predominate over the other deficiencies.[13] All energy is produced by means of enzymes, organic substances, whose principal component is protein. Vitamins are important only because they are part of certain enzymes. When protein is inadequate, however, none of the enzymes can be found in adequate quantities.[14] Under normal circumstances, the liver produces protein known as gamma globulins or anti-bodies, whose purpose is to combine with and make various harmless bacteria's, bacterial toxins and viruses. Therefore, its under-supply may encourage them, besides not allowing body fluids from becoming more acidic or alkaline or blood clotting. Protein mal-nutrition is found in all sections of population among the economically underdeveloped countries of the world.

In fact, the condition, particularly in its less acute form is now usually referred to as '*protein-caloric mal-nutrition*'. During the last few decades its wide, almost epidemic, explosive spreading has been noticed especially among the young children of developing countries. This metabolic-dietary diseases in infants and young children were known extensively studied in Europe, particularly in Germany in the first decade of 20th century. They are related to a greatly reduced protein, carbohydrates ration and were called 'starchy food dystrophy' occurring in dry (Marasmus) and in 'Edematous' forms which Cicely Williams termed *Kwashiorkor*.[15] These designations are still in use, but without the emphasis that both forms are based on an absolute protein intake usually far below the requirement. *Kwashiorkor* and *Marasmus* are a nutritional syndrome confined to the period of late breast feeding, weaning and post-weaning phases of the child's life due to deficiency of enough protective food like protein of high biological value, vitamins and other *substances* that would augment active growth. The word *Kwashiorkor* is the name given to the disease by Accre people of 'Gold Coast' and was introduced to the medical world in 1935 'the disease the child gets when the next baby is born, i.e. the sickness of the deposed child.[16] In countries with low economic standards like India, scarcity of fatty food in the market and old customs, fat intake of a large percentage of the population is usually low. Before completing weaning period, fat is available to young infants from the breast milk of the mother. Human milk is superior to any other milk due to presence of the essential *unstarched fatty acid*. That is why in many countries today breast feeding is on the decline and Marasmus show upward trend. Besides protein-caloric mal-nutrition, another disease often found in conjunction with protein-caloric mal-nutrition is Avitaminosis-A. This deficiency disease which in its most severe form, manifests itself by drying of the membranes of the eye (Xerophthalmia) and other changes (Keratomalacia) that cause destruction of the eye and total blindness occurs frequently but not constantly in association with protein-caloric mal-nutrition. The agent in this case is deficiency of vitamin-A, and the victim most frequently is the young pre-school child, though people of all ages may be affected. In India, about five million persons are visually handicapped and every fifth blind in the world is an Indian. Blindness in the majority of cases is due to mal-nutrition, or due to poor absorption of vitamin-A.[12] Its deficiency affects the skin before any organ. The skin becomes dry, rough, thick and scaly (Xeroderma). *Thiamine*, *Riboflavin* and *Niacin mal-nutrition*. Generally, Vitamin-B occurs together in food, no person can be deficient in any one of this group without being deficient in another. But there are degrees of variations as there are different individual. Formerly, the disease *Beri-Beri* was thought to be the result of thiamine deficiency and *Pellagra* due to lack of niacin. In fact, these diseases result from multiple deficiency of all the vitamins of this group, the lack of thiamine or niacin being only dominant. Its deficiency mainly affects tongue by fusing the taste buds and in severe cases it may be cut by grooves and fissures that it looks like a relief map of the grand canyon and surrounding territories. All these vitamins together related to energy metabolism and their requirement are directly related to energy expenditure.

Vitamin-C

The relationship of faulty diet to disease is an old story. James Lind's famous '*Treatise on Scurvy*' was published in 1753. What was new of the 1963 Nutritional Congress was the debate on dietary factors in the causation of *Cardiovascular* diseases.[18] Scurvy has played an important role in history. Survey shows that three-fourths of our population get less than the required quantity of vitamin-C. Vitamin-C helps to form and maintain a strong cement like material, known as *Collagen*, which holds together all the cells of the body and uses about one-third of all the body protein, except that the 'concrete' in healthy body is in the form of stiff jelly.[19] The base of the bones and of developing teeth given all these structure strength and elasticity. Its under-supply allows the tissues to break down and lack of calcium allows it to weaken against external agents.

Vatamin-D and Calcium

Nutrition is closely related to the normal processes of bone formation, growth and remodelling, for the skeleton is not a static unalterable structure. It is undisputed that vitamin-D aids the absorption of calcium, favours its retention and improves its utility. Besides, it relaxes nerves, induces sound sleep and decreases sensitivity to pain. While calcium helps in the transformation of nerve impulses, when difficult nerve becomes tense. Grouchy, wastage of energy etc. its under-supply become an air-swallower, indigestion coupled with insomnia and blood clotting. *Rickets* is a disease of those deprived of sources of vitamin–D of the sun-light and is more severe in those whose diet inadequate amount of calcium containing food, particularly milk.

Osteomalacia occurs in adult, particularly women during pregnancy and lactation, for during these times, mother's body must supply the essential nutrients for the child as well as for herself. Besides this, during lactation, women excrete more calcium, has been vividly described as with each child the condition takes a step forward as the body further drained of its minerals and vitamins. And with each child the condition becomes more piteous, the mother is more imprisoned in the house due to pain and deformities, her chances of earning more money, of getting more food and more sunlight are curtailed.[20]

Iron

Nutritional *anaemia* has been recognized for some time as a common deficiency state. It can be the result of inadequate protein, iodine, cobalt, copper, vitamin-E or due to any of the vitamin-B deficiency as every nutrient has a role in building healthy blood. Much anaemia does exist, however, which can be correlated with iron[21]. Iron, as a cause of nutritional anaemia, seems to be true in case of India and adjacent tropical countries.

In tropical countries, e.g. India, dietary intake generally ranges from 15 to 30 mg but the amount of available iron for absorption appears much less, poor absorption from food stuffs of vegetable origin. Therefore, it will be difficult to achieve a satisfactory level of iron ration in the population at large. Many factors like the decrease in physical activity and caloric intake, the change in man from hunting to agriculture pursuits and lastly, due to refinement in food preparation associated with decrease in contamination of iron and increase in activities such as phosphates and energy, vitamin-D, thiamine and vitamin-A have reduced the iron availability.

Iodine

A great amount of existing research has centred around iodine. In many mountainous regions of the world, especially in limestone areas, troubles with the thyroid gland have been endemic.[22] Endemic goitre is associated with an insufficiency of iodine in food and water.

Under-Nutrition

This form of mal-nutrition refers to the state of chronic under-nutrition and its full effect is probably immeasurable at the present moment. It has been the 'normal' state for so many years among a large section of the people in the world. Its physical effects vary with the victim according to age and condition.

A comparison of the food eaten in India and in other parts of the world clearly brings out the fact that our food is deficient in many respects. Indians eat more cereal than people in more developed countries and they eat far less of animal product than our counterparts. Thus, our food is short of animal protein and fats. An average Indian needs about 2400 calories per day to keep the body fit, but about 30 per cent gets less than 1700 calories; about 40 per cent gets between 1700-2300 calories and the remaining population gets more than this.[23] In case of other nutrients, situation is more pathetic. In general, Indian diets lack in more than one nutrient. This results in lethargic condition which is a common feature among the low income group people.

Diseases

The study of geography of diseases forms an important part of medical geography. It tries to analyse the environmental conditions coupled with other factors under which various categories of diseases spread. Geographical factors have far the most part only an indirect effect on the causation of diseases.

The discipline, which is associated with diseases like cholera, plague, typhoid, fever and small-pox is called 'Epidemiology' or may be defined as the ecology of the pathogenic organisms of communicable diseases in human society[24] and are the result of interaction between the pathogen and the human organism under specific environmental conditions.

On the basis of mode of their transmission, communicable diseases may be classified as follows[25]:

1. Oronasal
   (i) Tuberculosis
   (ii) Small-pox
   (iii) Chicken-pox
   (iv) Measles
   (v) Diphtheria

2. Orofecal
   (i) Diarrhoea and Dysentery
   (ii) Cholera
   (iii) Typhoid
   (iv) Food Poisoning
   (v) Infective Hepatitis
   (vi) Poliomyelitis

3. Soil Transmitted Diseases
   (i) Round Worm
   (ii) Hook Worm
   (iii) Trichuris Trichura
   (iv) Tetanus

4. Skin Contact
   (i) Leprosy
   (ii) Scabies
   (iii) Genetal Contact V.D.

5. Arthropods
   (i) Malaria
   (ii) Filaria
   (iii) Dengue fever
   (iv) Yellow fever

6. Zoonoses
   (i) Brucellosis
   (ii) Rabies
   (iii) Plague

7. Miscellaneous
    (i) Trachoma
    (ii) Blindness
    (iii) Tracontiasis

Besides communicable diseases, there are other types of diseases which take a toll of human life annually. Among others, the author is presently concerned with nutritional deficiency diseases. According to J.M. May(1961), who worked on the ecology of mal-nutrition, most forms of mal-nutrition or under-nutrition are caused by deficiency of some essential nutrients either in quantity or quality of food taken by an individual with the result that certain deficiency diseases occur. The main deficiency diseases prevalent in the country are, *Kwashiorkor, Marasmus, Avitaminosis-A (Xerophthalmia), Keratomalacia, (Nightblindness). Beri-Beri, Pellagra, Ariboflavinosis, Anaemia, Scurvy, Rickets, Osteomalacia, Goitre* etc.

Kwashiorkor: Kwashiorkor appears to be a multiple deficiency syndrome (niacin, riboflavin, protein etc.). Its first symptoms are marked by irritability, attacks of diarrhoea and light swelling of wrists, hands and feet. The skin of the entire body loses its gloss and becomes reddish or muddy.[26]

It is difficult to give the spatial distribution of it due to its different names in different parts of the world. According to Trowell (1949), it is widely distributed in tropical Africa, India, Sri Lanka, Malaysia, Indo-China, Java, Cuba, Central America and Southern Brazil.[27] In South India, for example, a survey was carried out in four states, where 85 per cent of the population live in small rural villages and have monthly income of less than 500 rupees. Here about one per cent of the children aged, 1-5 years showed signs of Kwashiorkor.[28] In addition, for everyone case of it, two cases of *marasmus* 3-5 cases of vitamin deficiency and five of *anaemia* were found (Fig 3.1).

Marasmus : It differs from kwashiorkor in various ways, the marasmic child is wasted not swollen. His hair is dull and dry, but not discoloured. He has thin and wrinkled skin with lost elasticity, but does not breakdown. The child does not refuse food and shows less resentment unlike kwashiorkor. Terrible wasting make the eye look enormous and starting etc. Why marasmus develops instead of kwashiorkor is not clearly understood.

Avitaminos: This deficiency disease which in its most severe form manifests itself by drying one of the membranes of the eye. There is

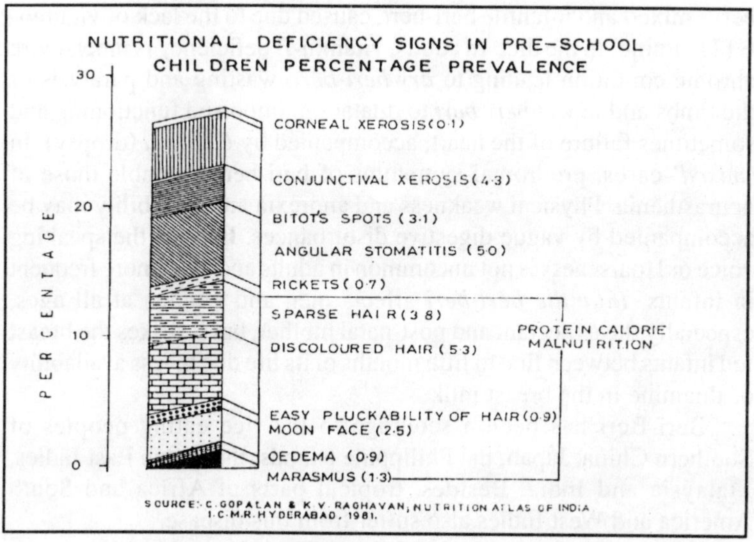

Fig. 3.1 : Nutritional deficiency Signs in Per-School Children Percentage Prevalence

general agreement that dryness of the conjuctiva which is called *Xerosis* or *Xerophthalmia* is a common symptom of vitamin-A deficiency. Whitish foamy patches (Bitot's spots) may appear and ulceration, infection can ensue. Photophobia has been noted in some cases. *Keratomalacia* brings certain changes that cause destruction of the eye and may lead to total blindness. Keratotic follicular lesions of the skin (Phrynoderma) apparently can be caused by deficiency of either vitamin-A or vitamin-C, but the latter results in hoemorrage, because of vitamin-C deficiency. It may be the results of severe dysentery coupled with less elements of vitamin-B complex. Defective dark adaptation (night-blindness) is generally thought to be a very common, an early sign of vitamin-A deficiency. 'Kruse', believed that Xerosis may precede the development of night-blindness.[29] According to passmore, Xerophthalmia and Keratomalacia is probably the most frequent sign of mal-nutrition which occurs in India.[30] The victims are frequently the young pre-school children, though people of any age may be affected. The children of South India, Sri Lanka, Burma (Myanmar), Malaysia and above all Indonesia are those most stricken.

Beri-Beri : It is usually recognized as 'dry beri-beri', 'wet beri-

beri', mixed and infantile beri-beri, caused due to the lack of vitamin-B (Thiamine) in the diet. In adults, vitamin-B deficiency is much more chronic condition leading to *dry beri-beri*, wasting and paralysis of the limbs and in *wet beri-beri* to dilatation, impoised functioning and sometimes failure of the heart, accompanied by *Oedema* (dropsy). In '*mixed*' cases, prodromal symptoms of beri-beri resemble those of neurasthenia. Physical weakness and anorexia and irritability may be accompanied by vague digestive disturbances. Loss of the speaking voice or Hoarseness is not uncommon in adults and even more frequent in infants. *Infantile beri-beri* affects men and women at all ages, especially the expectant and post-natal mother, but it strikes the breast fed infants between first to fifth months of its life due to less availability of thiamine in the breast milk.

Beri-Beri has been a scourage to the rice eating peoples of Southern China, Japan, the Philippine Islands, the Dutch East Indies, Malaysia and India. Besides, tropical parts of Africa and South America and West Indies also suffer from this disease.[31]

Pellagra : It is not sharply defined. The principal manifestations of the disease in the advanced stage are of several kinds, viz. a dermatitis having special features, digestive disorders, degenerative lesions of the spinal cord and psychoses of the confusional type. The syndrome is ascribed principally to deficiency of niacin and partly to deficiency of other elements of the heat stable portion of the vitamin-B complex.

Data on the world distribution of pellagra were compiled and tabulated by Sobrell (1943). The data then and still available is far from complete. Sporadic cases of pellagra may appear almost everywhere in the world.[32] Pellagra is common in the Bombay presidency and the increasing recognition indicates that the disease is fairly common in India.[33]

Ariboflavinosis: It is found generally among maize eaters like pellagra but also in communities with staple rice diet. It is somewhat like pellagra, but the more characteristics signs attributed to it are ocular signs and symptoms like itching, burning and a sense of roughness of the lids combined with mild photophobia (dimness of vision in poor light and partial blindness are less frequent), angular stomatitis (by fissures at the angles of mouth). The lips may be abnormally red, cracked and scaling (particularly lower lips) coupled with lethargy, mental tension, depression, retardation etc., due to the deficient amount of niacin in diet.

Like pellagra, this is found all over the world. In India signs of ariboflavinosis have been observed by Aykroyd and others (1942). The diseases is common in South India.[34] Thomson and Freeman (1947) described an outbreak of it in Indian soldiers on the north-west frontier.[35]

Anaemia : Due to continued deficiency of either iron or protein in the diet, the reserves and adaptation mechanisms are unable to maintain the level of circulating hemoglobin within normal limits. The resulting fall in the hemoglobin concentration and oxygen-carrying of the blood, produces the condition of Anaemia. Nutritional anaemia caused by dietary deficiency or by failure to absorb substances essential for nutrition, fall into three principal categories, viz., the hypochromic, the macrocytic and the dimorphic or mixed type.

Microcytic anaemia, which were regarded as essentially of nutritional origin have been seen in Bombay by Wills,[36] in Calcutta by Napier and by Edwards in Assam.[37] Many of the cases occurred in pregnant women. Other cases were observed by Taylor and Chuttani in Indian males, particularly vegetarian.[38] The other two types of anaemia are not of nutritional origin.

Scurvy : Scurvy is characterized by increasing weekness, lethargy accompanied by irritability, dizziness, loss of appetite and craving for salt. In latter stages hoemorrhage is noticed into skin and subcutaneous tissues. Dryness of the skin is also common with spongy bleeding purplish gums. Sporadic cases of scurvy in infants or adults may be encountered in India and such cases have been numerous during the times of food scarcity.

Rickets and Osteomalacia: Rickets is known as 'English disease.[39] It is a disease that is caused due to lack of vitamin-D. It affects not only legs and hands but also the pelvic and chest region may become malformed.

In rickets there is a failure to deposit calcium and phosphorus in the growing bones. Corresponding diseases in the case of adults called *Osteomalacia*, the bones soften due to withdrawal and excretion of the deposited calcium and phosphorus in the body. It is common in pregnant women, who get less sun-shine. In the past, rickets was thought to be rare in tropical countries due to environment asset. The disease is more frequent in urban areas than in the rural settings. In Calcutta and Bombay, children showing signs of rickets have been seen. One area in Kangra valley in the Himachal Pradesh is unique in India in having an unusually high prevalence of rickets (56 per cent of 156 children examined). The average figure for other parts of India being between 0.2 and 3.2 per cent[40]. Osteomalacia is found almost in many parts of India.

Goitre : As old as history itself is the incidence of *Goitre* in the human race. Enlargement of thyroid glands result due to long term deficient supply of iodine. When the iodine supply is very low even the enlarged gland cannot produce enough thyroxin, the energy metabolism will be slowed down. The person become sluggish and very sensitive to cold, the muscles become flabby and the mental processes are also slowed down. It is quite different from other deficiency diseases so far described, as it is neither confined to the developing nations in the tropical and sub-tropical regions nor to the population suffering from poverty. Mountainous and sub-mountainous regions—the Himalayas, the Alps and the Andes—the classical sites where endemic goitre is found. It also occurs in the plains and even along coastal regions. It has been estimated that there are some 300 million people suffering from goitre in the world.

REFERENCES

1. Schifferes, J.J., *Healthier Living*, Sixth International Congress of Nutrition in Retrospect, New York, 1965, p. 94.
2. Barker, G., *Health in Independent India*: New Delhi, 1957, pp. 125-26.
3. Pyke, M., *Nutrition*, New York, 1961, p. 20.
4. *Report of the Health Survey and Development Committee*, Vol. II, New Delhi, 1946, p. 69.
5. *The Times of India*, New Delhi, April 7, 1978, p. 2.
6. *Report of the Health Survey and Development Committee*, *op. cit.*, p. 69.
7. W.H.O., *Mal-Nutrition and Disease*, Geneva, 1963, p. 3.
8. Maxim, E., Dixitt, M.C. and Mudambi, *Human Nutrition* Principal and Application in India, New Delhi.
9. May, J.M., *The Ecology of Mal-nutrition in the Far and Near East*, New York, 1961, p. 22.
10. Corwin, E.H.L., *Ecology of Health*, New York, 1949, p. 55.
11. Sukhatme, P.V., *Feeding India's Growing Millions*, Bombay, 1965, p. 57.
12. Chandra, P., Non-nutritional Cause of Mal-nutrition, *The Ind. J. Nutri. and Diete.*, Coimbatore, 1975, p. 168.
13. Davis, A., *Let's Eat Right to Keep Fit*, London, 1971, p. 20.
14. *Ibid.*, p. 20.
15. Gyorgy, P., Rajammal, P., Devadas and Chandra Shekhar, U., 'Calories in the Treatment of Protein-Caloric Mal-nutrition', *The Ind. J. of Nutri, and Diete.*, Coimbatore, 1973, No. 5, p. 252.

16. Krishna-Murthy, C.S., '*Mal-nutrition in Infants and A Deficiency Disease*', National Health Seminar, Madras, 1965, p. 52.
17. Tahiliani, B., '*Vitamin-A Deficiency' A Common Cause of Blindness, Carvan*, May (i), New Delhi 1975, p. 48.
18. Schifferes, J.J., *op. cit.*, p. 95.
19. Davis, A., op. cit., p. 123.
20. Bicknell, F. and Prescott, F., '*The Vitamins in Medicine*', London, 1953, p. 35.
21. Davis, A., *op. cit.*, p. 177.
22. Mottram, V.H., '*Human Nutrition*', Londan, 1963, p. 27
23. Misra, R.P., '*Medical Geography of India*'. New Delhi, 1970, p. 159.
24. Zhdanov, V., '*Epidemiology*', Moscow, pp. 7-8
25. Jerath, B.K., *Synopsis of Social and Preventive Medicine*, Ludhiana, 1970, p. 71.
26. Shattuck, G.C., *Diseases of the Tropics*, New York 1951, p. 692.
27. Trowell, H.C., 'Malignant Mal-nutrition' (Kwashiorkor), *Tr. Roy. Soc. Trop. Med. and Hyg.* 1946, pp. 39-437.
28. Rao, S.K., Swaminathan, M.C., Swarup, S. and Patwardhan, *V.N.*, 'Protein Mal-nutrition in South India', *Bull. World Heath Organisation* (20), 1959, p. 603.
29. Kruse, H.D., 'Medical Evaluation of Nutritional Status', *Pub. Health Rep., Washington* D.C. 1941, IV, 56: 1301
30. Passmore, R., 'Mixed Deficiency Diseases in India', *Tr. Roy. Soc. Trop. Med. and Hyg.* 1947, 41 : p. 189.
31. Shattuck, G.C., op. cit., p. 650.
32. Sobrell, W.H., '*Nutrition in Preventive Medicine', A Hand Book of Nutrition*, American Medical Association, 1943, p. 475.
33. Stannus, H.S., 'Pellagra and Pellagra like Conditions in warm Climates', *Trop Diseases Bull.*, 1936, 33: p. 729.
34. Aykroyd, W.R., Verma, O.P., 'Superficial Keratitis due to Riboflavin Deficiency' *Indian Medical Gazetteer*, Delhi 1942, 77; p.1.
35. Thomson, A.M. and Freeman, B., 'An Epidemic of Riboflavin Deficiency in Indian Troops', *Tr. Roy. Soc. Trop. Med. and Hyg.*, 1947, 40 :399.
36. Wills, L., 'Pernicious Anaemia, Nutritional Microcytic Anaemia and Tropical Sprue Blood'. *Ind. J. Med. Res.* 1948, 3: 36.
37. Napier, L.E. and Edward, M., 'Anaemia in Pregnancy in Calcutta'. *Ind. J. Med. Res.,* 1941, No. 33.
38. Taylor, G.F. and Chuttani, P.N., 'Nutritional Microcytic Anaemia and the Animal Protein of Diet', *Brif. Med. Jour.*, 1945, 1:800.
39. Taylor, C.M. and Pye, O.F., *Foundation of Nutrition*, New York, 1966, p. 248.
40. Patwardhan, V.N., 'Nutrition in India', *Ind. J. of Med. Soc.,* 1962, p. 343.

4 Environment and Health

Natural environment plays an important role in controlling the health of human beings. Its effect is very often felt through air and water. Pollution of any one of these may result in the spread of various diseases. Impurities and lack of certain nutrients in the drinking water may lead to deficiency diseases. The other elements of natural environment are equally important and have their effect on the human health.

Every character is subject to two types of effect and what is more explanatory is that genetic and environmental agencies may produce variations, which cannot be distinguished from one another by inspection. The individual may develop poorly because of inadequate nutrition or due to poor genes and only appropriate observations of relations on different planes of nutrition can finally distinguish these causes.[1] While it is true that in a formal sense each of us may be regarded as reflecting the influence of the genes he bears and of the environment in which he has developed, that environment has certain peculiarity depending on his family and the community or society to which he belongs. These will altogether determine to a great extent not only his physical environment, but also the education he receives, the ideas he imbibes, the convention or customs to which he will conform (or against which he will rebel) and the activities he will pursue.

Human characters and characteristics are affected by the environment. Each of us requires from his environment food stuffs of an appropriate kind and shelter. The effects of change in these environmental agencies are too striking and too well known. With the discovery of vitamins, the elucidation of dietic needs and improvement in the availability of food supplies, the nutritional status of the population especially in western countries, where health is better, deficiency diseases are rare and the rate of growth is higher. In contrast, the case of some of the Asian countries may be quoted, where the people are still living at a bare level of subsistence and whose physique and rate of growth display their low nutritional status. Improvement in nutrition has been accompanied by similar changes in general standards of clothing and housing, as well as in the development of adequate level of sanitation. The success in improvement in nutrition, housing and the control of diseases brings its own problems. The immediate effect of these measures is the reduction in the death rate. Then, unless the birth rate falls correspondingly, there must inevitably be a rise in total population. Our improvements in nutrition, housing and the control of disease have upset the biological balance upon which depends population size. We must expect man to show some genetical diversity in disease resistance and we have, in fact, direct evidence that relation tends to resemble one another in their resistance or susceptibility to disease.

In general, however, the variety, diversity, intensity and geographical spread of environmental change by man is accelerating and as problems of pesticide contamination, climatic change or water pollution, mal and under-nutrition worsen, they demand our attention. The greatest, but still only partial, exception to this situation are found in the fields of ecology and physical geography. Ecology as defined by many advocates is the science of man and environment and tries to study the relationship between organisms and their environments. Geography, on the other hand, studies the relationship between man and his environment with emphasis on the spatial manifestations of this relationship. Unlike ecologists, geographers have tended to study broad spatial patterns and relations between man and landscape. But the tradition of considering man's influence and of relating numerous varied aspects of the environment to one another are longstanding, going back to the works of Alexander Von Humboldt and Karl Ritter, early in the nineteenth century.

Geographers should provide the emerging science of environment with an appreciation of scales and maps and valuable methods of analysis as well as the integrative interdisciplinary view points mentioned above. The contributions of other sciences have generally been limited in their approach. It can, therefore, be said that in the study of environment, geography is as important as any other natural sciences.

In a historic sense, there is little that is new, though perhaps something is be considered in the concept of a casual relationship between the environment in which man lives and the state of his health.

The German physician Alfred Grot John wrote early in the last century that social conditions (a) may create or favour a predisposition for a disease, (b) may themselves cause disease directly, (c) may transmit the causes of disease and (d) may influence the course of a disease.[2] (A) There is enough evidence that mal-nutrition, extreme fatigue and exposure to cold and dampness are among the conditions that may create or favour a predisposition for a disease. (B) Occupational diseases and accidents are some among a large group of illness that may be traced quite directly to the causative force, wholly or in part, of social conditions. (C) The so called crowding and filth, education, income, may result or influence the course of a disease.

Environment appears to affect man in two ways. It may reach man and affect his health; it may act upon or within his body as a material agent or upon his mind and emotions as a non-material agent, although sooner or later this very well produces a material effect[3] factor's affecting human health.

Disease is a multiple phenomenon which occurs only if various factors coincide in time and space. We have to study the relationship between them—the pathological factors and the geographical factors, which have been termed as *pathogens* and *geogens* by May.[4] Some of the relationships are well known, but many have not been yet explored fully.

Pathological factors :

(a) Causative agents
(b) Vectors
(c) Intermediate hosts
(d) Reservoirs
(e) Man.

Geographical factors :

(a) Physical (climate, latitude, rainfall, humidity, temperature, pressure, sun-shine, clouds, wind and its direction, velocity, radiation, relief, soil and hydrology).
(b) Human and social or socio-cultural (population distribution and density), standard of living, housing, diet, clothing, sanitation, income, communication, religion, and superstition, drug addiction.

(c) Biological (vegetable life, animal life on earth and water, parasitism, human and animal prevalent diseases, dominal blood groups).

Many writers have focused their attention and tried to establish and illustrate the relationship between the man's health and his environment under different headings (e.g. material and non-material environment, biotic community and ecosystem, relationship between pathogens and geogens etc.). The human group must be considered in stable equilibrium not merely with reference to temperature, humidity, sun-shine, altitude etc., but also to their indirect effects, the interwoven chain of biotic communities to which it is inextricably linked the plants it cultivates, the animals it breeds and even the insects which are indigenous to the region.[5]

Human diseases can be said to be the net result of the "convergence in time and space within the person of the patient of environment stimuli, organic, inorganic or socio-cultural. These stimuli are a challenge which includes a tissular response, that is, disease (communicable, degenerative or behavioural) which in turn eventually results in ecologic adaptation and survival or in total maladjustment and death".[6] Disease is thus "that alteration of the living tissues which jeopardizes survival in their environment and which results from an accidental collision between two or more forms of life, each pursuing its own destiny".[7]

The two forms of life which collide with each other to create human diseases are human beings and pathological factors (causative or organic agent, viruses, rickettsias, spirochetes, bacteria, fungi, protozoa and metazoa), causing disease, their nature is still under discussion. A definite correlation seems to exist between a number of these viruses and temperature and humidity. It has been noticed that the low temperature delays the onset of epidemics of sand-fly fever in India, whereas early warm weather usually accelerates outbreaks.

Spell of cold weather might affect the course of epidemics, it acts on both, vector and virus, but experiments proved that exposure to high temperatures may hasten the multiplication of the viruses of jungle yellow fever, in the mosquito. *Rickettsias* and the living organisms, completely parasitic, cannot exist outside living cells and can be differentiated in these main geographical groups, linked with ticks (North America and Brazil, South Africa, Asiatic groups, etc.) closely linked with mili-borne infections (Japan, South Asia, etc.) third group, more widespread is found in Europe and Central Asia is linked with fleas and lice, former causing epidemics and the latter epidemic typhus.

Spirochetes, are found worldwide but certain species seem to have definite geographical associations, some live in blood of man, transmitted by the bite of lice or ticks, another group passes directly from rodents, when man ingests food or water contaminated with the urine of an infected animal (jaundice infection). Next group needs rat bite (rat bite fever).

Bacteria are a vegetable origin comprising a large number of agents of human diseases, throughout the world (endemic and epidemic). Cholera has been observed all over the world in an epidemic form. But endemic foci of cholera from which epidemics spread out are few, limited to certain spots in India and possibly in China.

Fungi are group of plants related to bacteria, their existence is governed by various factors, e.g. humidity and temperature, a correlation that may explain their geographical distribution.

Protozoa and *Metazoa* are also subject to geographical condition that favours their development. Protozoa are a large group of unicellular animals, cause most widespread tropical diseases, e.g. malaria (whose causative agent, a plasmodumin, is dependent on both man and mosquito for its existence) and *amoebic* dysentery etc. Metazoa are more complicated. They grow to be visible to naked eyes and comprise all the helminthes that inhabit the tissues, the bowels (as carides, hook worms), the circulatory system (schistosomes, filaria) and the viscera (liver flunkes etc.) of man. Their eggs need certain soil conditions to hatch, intermediate hosts to develop the larva and certain vectors and circumstances to reach their permanent hosts. All these stages are subject to powerful geographical influences.

Vectors

The life and activity of these vectors are also the subject of geographical influence, e.g. *Glossina palpalis*, for instance the most important vectors of African sleeping sickness, require a relatively dense wood or thicket of a more or less evergreen type and the larva need a certain kind of sand in which they develop. In the same way, species of anopheline mosquitoes require various breeding habitants (fresh or saline water, water in the cells holes). The causative agents reach man in various ways, directly or indirectly. Some attack through respiratory passages, e.g. viruses of measles, mumps, smallpox and the respiratory diseases. Others are swallowed with food, as in cholera, typhoid fever, amoebic dysentery; next, through skin as in ancylostomiasis. Other may transfer the germs superficially (flies, cockroaches, beetles etc.).

Intermediate hosts enter into the pathological complex as a part of organism essential to the lifecycle of the agent (human flunke infections, broad tape worm etc.). Next to this comes the *Reservoirs* and carry on the infection in nature, when man is unavoidable or suitably protected and also as supplement to man. Agent spends parts of his life in the cycle, until picked up by the vectors, sometimes expelled by the host. Lastly, comes the man as a pathogen and works an infection carrier.

Geographical Factors Affecting Health

The various geographical factors should be correlated individually with the human health and diseases. Health is often defined as a state in which the mental and physical activities of the body are adjusted satisfactorily to the environment. It is said that they are influenced by two aspects—firstly, nature (inheritance) and secondly, nature (environment). Therefore, disease which is the result of disturbed equilibrium, between external (biological, physical, and socio-cultural) and internal forces is caused by the interaction of patient, agent (causative organisms) and the environment. So it is clear that maladjustment of a person to his environment may lead to ill health. Here, geographical environment does not mean only the physical conditions of any particular place, but it includes totality of the environment as indicated here.

A. *Physical Environment* (inorganic): Topography-upland, lowland and climate—excessive rainfall—and extreme weather conditions.
B. *Socio-cultural Environment*: Population distribution and density, standard of living, housing, diet agricultural production, holdings, government policies, clothing, sanitation, income, communication, religious customs and superstitions, drug addictions.
C. *Biological Environment* : Vegetable life, animal life on earth and water, parasitism—human and animal, prevalent diseases, dominant blood groups etc.

A. *Physical Environment*

Environmental factors with a possible effects on man can be classified as stable factors of the natural environment, which are not subject to major change, e.g. solar constant, gravitation, the composition of atmosphere, relief, climatic conditions, the general order of magnitude of temperature etc. These factors determine the conditions of phylogenesis, the mechanism of morpho-physiologic adaptations, that is the connection with the external environment in general. The main periodically changing environmental factors include the seasons of the year, hours of the day. The secondary variables include seasonal and *diurnal* changes in atmospheric conditions. These factors are reflected in the rhythm of life of living things.

From the environment a human being needs certain chemicals, e.g. vitamins, proteins, minerals and other substances are neutral in their effect on the physiology of man. At the same time, a beneficial-substance may become detrimental depending upon the amount. All of these inorganic factors challenge in many ways the living cells, ability to cope with the environment.

Among the inorganic factors which affect health of man, topography has a relatively indirect influence. Topography includes all the characteristics which give a piece of land its individuality in terms of elevation, relief, scope, rock types, soils and minerals and water contents. To a considerable extent, topography determines the capacity of an area to produce things needed for the survival of all living things, including the viruses which cause diseases. Areas having plains formed by rivers are good to produce many crops; mountain areas produce less as they have less extensive level lands with good soils.

Relief has bearing on the onset and end of several epidemics in an area. It is often noted that cholera ends with the onset of rains in well drained areas. Malaria is common where relief provides opportunity for water to stagnate.

A detailed study of different categories of soils has led scientists to believe that there is a close relationship between soil, human nutrition and health. The healthy growth of food plant is very much determined by the presence of required mineral constituents in the soil. Soils which lack in essential mineral constituents lead to poor growth of the plants and thus human beings are deprived of the essential nutrients from the poor crop grown in poor soil.[8] Whenever we think about the problem of food supply, we cannot but think of soil. It is the soil that determines not only what we shall eat, but whether we shall eat at all.[9] The key to successful operation of the cultivator lies in the balance between energy input and production of food stuffs or energy output. As man cultivates the soil, plants and weeds the crops, he is providing inputs of energy for this system, which operates through the medium of land. Concurrently, the system is receiving energy in the form of sun-shine and rainfall, which operates through the medium of land. The combined energy inputs result in an energy output from the land which is available to the agriculturist in the form of food and this output must at least be equal to man's energy input plus conversion losses, if the system is to be self-perpetuating. There may be considerable energy losses, for man does not devote the whole of his available energy to cultivation. Likewise, all energy inputs do not result in the growth of food.

Assuming natural energy inputs to be constant in any locality, man's ability to derive sufficient energy from the land depends upon two factors, his own energy inputs (the actual magnitude of energy inputs is important only in that is must be exceeded by the energy outputs, i.e. food, which constitutes his future energy supplies), and the ability of the land to convert the supplies of energy to food stuffs, which will vary directly with fertility factors and agricultural techniques.[10]

The importance of soil to man lies in its functions as a reservoir of nutrients and as a medium of nutrient exchange.[11] These nutrients, which include air and water are essential for plant growth. Any action that impedes or prevents the provision of useful soil nutrients to crops is detrimental to agriculture.

Soil which lacks in certain essential food elements may cause some diseases, e.g. Goitre, Tetanus, Gangrene. They produce (Bacterias, Parasites) diseases, when they gain access to wounds of the body.[12] Unlike most of the deficiency diseases, the occurrence of endemic goitre is not determined by socio-cultural factors, rather by the nature of water, soil and its content of iodine.[13]

Climate generally signifies the combined effects of the sun, the atmosphere, and the earth on the biotic phenomena including human life. Its chief elements are air, temperature, pressure, humidity precipitation (rain, snow or other forms) etc. The combined effect of all these is modified by local conditions, e.g. distribution of land and water, altitude, latitude, etc.

The influence of climate is felt by all of us at all times. Several studies show a sort of direct relationship between climate and the physical and the mental vitality of man.[14] One of the findings brings out energy differences between the races living in warm and temperate climates, which cannot be explained by differences in diet and mode of living alone. 'The man in the tropics has a lower oxygen consumption, a lower blood pressure and a lower capacity to meet emergencies than the inhabitants of the temperate zones.[15]

Some psychologists even feel that each climate gives rise to a mentality which is characteristically its own. Several diseases are linked directly or indirectly with climate. Moreover, the climatic conditions when marked by a monotony of seasons, as we see in the tropical and sub-tropical conditions, lead to a life-pattern which does not prepare human beings to adapt themselves to changes. Then again, the influence of climate on the diet of the people is far reaching.

The climatic conditions are no doubt of primary importance in determining the distribution of human energy, since the climate of a region determines more than any other single factor, not only the health of a people but also the type and fertility of the soil and its economic utilization.[16] In predominantly agricultural countries, like India, climate determines to a great extent, the amount and nature of food available to people. If the rains are good, people have more and better food to eat, and if it fails, famines occur and people suffer from both under and mal-nutrition.

It has long been recognized that the geographical selectivity of diseases like Pellagra and Beri-Beri is due to crop popularity and the dietary customs of the population. More, recently other physiological effects have also been associated with poor nutritional habits. However, variations in the nutritional status of people living in different areas and climate may not be entirely due to improper food selection but partially to the vitamin content of supposedly adequate diet. The climate effects on thiamine content of meat is also proved. There is a great deft of thiamine in Panama meats, and the investigators who ate the native meat noted that the output of thiamine in their urine decreased steadily. As soon as they ate ham imported from Argentina or United States, the thiamine excretion levels were raised. So, animal proteins are by and large the most deficient element in our food. Moist climates are not favourable for animal growth, nor are they too arid and dry ones. In the moist climates the quality of the animals is poor even though there is an abundance of green fodder and grazing grounds. Disease takes a heavy toll of life there and yield of milk and meat per animal is very low.

Climatic influence on health is not only indirect. Higher temperatures and humidity tend to reduce working efficiency of man and strain the physiological conditions of our body. The best climate is that in which heat losses are balanced by heat production in the body without much strain. Climates which are too cold or too hot are, therefore, not satisfactory. But a person can normally adjust himself except when he is too young, old or sick. The process of acclimatization to heat consists largely in leaving to sweat more volume with less salt content, and this must be accompanied by taking more water and more salt.[17]

In the tropical climates, there seems to be a lowering of blood pressure, the volume of blood presumably increases, but it is more diluted, sweating takes a toll of plasma, fluid and salts which must be made up. There is decreases in gastric secretions, accompanied by constipation and impaired appetite and digestion; there is also reduced energy for work, but this may often be a sign of mal-nutrition or some other trouble. Hence, those who have a higher energy production because of an overactive thyroid are likely to become neurasthenic in the tropics. There is less oxygen per cubic metre in hot than in cold air, and this may reduce the effectiveness of all bodily functions unless the body becomes adjusted to it. Constant sweating and the increase of blood flow to the capillaries induced by warmth have a harmful effect in blood chemistry, and the tone of internal organs, lowering resistance to infection.[18] Excessive heat tends to exhaust the people and create heat strokes.

Cold with reference to its severity increases the caloric requirements, high carbohydrate diets with top heavy protein to improve tolerance, but in hot environment energy requirement decreases as compared to temperate climate due to a diminished basal expenditure of energy or to greater deficiency in certain types of muscular work associated with lighter clothing or to a lessened capacity for work and less motivation or to all three. Water requirements are definitely increased, when sweating is included and somewhat in proportion to the amount of sweat secreted. During intense sweating thirst is not an adequate guide to water requirements. Salt requirements also increase, small losses in vitamins in the heat may increase slightly due to losses in minerals in the sweat and in the case of calcium, to fairly consistent increases in fecal losses in a hot environment, man's requirement for iron, and loss certainly for calcium may be increased in tropical environment.

The geographical differential which is most likely to suggest itself, particularly in a discussion of the variations in disease between warmer and cooler regions, is climate. The possibility that climate is an etiological agent of disease has been the matter of interest since the time of Hippocrates. It is not possible to test the specific relationship between climate and disease in a laboratory, but may be analysed with regard to difference in the prevalence of certain diseases in a particular geographical area.

It is said that not only does the lower metabolic level of people living in warm climates make them more susceptible to disease than those in temperate zones, but the variation in mental alertness also plays an important part in the geographical distribution of diseases—parasitic and infectious and mal-nutrition are their greater disease problems.

On the basis of studies made so far, it can be said that there is a rather close relationship between changes in the weather and certain diseases, e.g. common cold, pneumonia, infantile paralysis, cholera, smallpox, dysentery, etc. The greatest number of common cold occurs in winter while the cases of infantile paralysis, cholera and smallpox are maximum in the summer months. A close relationship is thus found between changes in the weather and acute respiratory and rheumatic infection. Impurities in the atmosphere also increase the susceptibility to infections.

It really matters little whether climate is directly responsible for the occurrence of a variety of infectious diseases or not, what is important is the fact that such diseases do exist, and they exist in tropical climates more than elsewhere. It is also important to note that the widespread incidence of debilitating, incapacitating, and life-shortening disease must seriously reduce both the desire for work and the efficiency of performance, and that these effects will, in turn, increase the likelihood of mal-nutrition and decrease the efficacy of preventive measure in a self-perpetuating cycle of poverty and disease.[19]

B. *Socio-Cultural Environment*

In the foregoing pages the influence of natural environment on the health of the people has been discussed. In this chapter author intends to study the influence of socio-cultural factors on health. The importance of these factors in matters of health has been recognized recently. A study of the interaction between human, socio-cultural environment and health is specially important in the under-developed countries like India, for people in countries characterized by a slow rate of change have adopted certain traditional lines. What often appears to be a dogged adherence of conservative people to harmful ways is not pure stubbornness—it is just that the new changes advocated do not make sense to them. There can be no escape from facing and solving the cultural equation of medicine, health, illness and treatment.[20]

The term socio-cultural as used here includes population, its density, standard of living, income, housing, food habits, agriculture, size of holding, government, policies, clothing, sanitation, communication, religious and social customs—values, beliefs, practices, superstitions and drug addictions. In a country like India where a great majority of the people live in rural areas, Indian culture may be termed as rural culture.

Man, being a social organism, is subject to complex social and economic order. It is equally essential for him to adjust himself to non-social surroundings, and it is due to mal-adjustment to social and non-social environment that many diseases are born. Abnormal demand often affects physiological system as well as organic relationships of the primary group and the rhythm of social routine that moulded and shaped his mental development for successive generations, prior to the present industrial age. Therefore, an optimum relationship between the rhythm of life and the rhythm of machine as well as the tempo of work has to be established for the safety and stability of the man'.[21]

Disease has been defined as mal-adjustment of living cells to their environment. It is for us to see how challenges arise from the environment and how the factors controlling the responses to those challenges in individual and in groups react. There is an important aspect of this reaction, challenge *versus* response that has not been considered, i.e. the circumstances that bring together the challenger and that challenged, stimulus and the response, disease and the host. It is realized that when man is concerned these intermediate factors that either being together or keep apart stimulus and individuals are summed up in the word 'socio-culture'. Socio-cultural factors are defined as the sum total of the concepts and techniques that human groups use and abide by in the environment in which they are placed in order to survive.

Socio-cultural factors influence disease occurrence in three main ways :

(i) By linking or separating challenges of the environment and host,
(ii) By challenging the environment,
(iii) By challenging the host population.

1. By linking and separating challenges and host, people built their houses with the material supported the environment, dress with the material procured from the nearest market and the cheapest place, eat the diet, the soil under their feet yields when treated by the techniques they know. They believe what their parents believed to be true. Then they transmit to their offsprings their way of life and this becomes part of their culture. Does it mean that a given culture at a given point is a best method for survival? Under changing circumstances it may even become detrimental. From the type of housing they are forced to adopt they get their plague and typhus and from the food which the soil, temperature and rain produce their protein deficiency. The relationships between socio-cultural factors and diseases are worth-noting.
2. Cultural influence disease pattern bringing about environment changes; building a dam for irrigation and canals for drainage, erecting houses, planting rice adding pesticides/gypsum to the water, all such changes carry with them host of inter-locked reactions.
3. Finally, cultural circumstances bring about changes in population genetic make up, thus changing the response of tissues to environmental changes. New agricultural techniques were developed.

It is axiomatic that at the present population level, more people means more environmental problems. According to experts, the earth's ultimate 'carrying capacity' or ability to support man is probably 30 billion people, but at a level of near starvation for the great majority. However, the distribution of food and other resources is uneven and hence widespread famine appears imminent.[22] With a total population of over one billion, India is the second largest country of the world. The absolute growth of population in the country is so high that India adds to its population the equivalent of a town of almost 20,000 inhabitants everyday. If this increase continues, there will be 900 million people by 1991 and a clear 1,000 million by 2000 A.D., this proved to be true as we are above 1 billion.

The alarming decennial growth rate of population, +25.5 in Uttar Pradesh, +27.6 and +24.7 in the districts of Faizabad and Sultanpur respectively, poses serious problems for social and economic development. It nullifies all efforts to improve the admittedly low standard of living of the people. The plans to increase the production of food and other commodities and to improve the services through welfare measures are either deferred or frustrated, because the increasing population overtakes the increase in agricultural productivity as also the improvement in education, public health, sanitation, etc.

Many of the problems like under-employment, subdivision of holdings, lack of capital, and indebtedness occur together in under-developed countries, that is the condition in which any further increase in population will result in a decrease in the income level. Malthus first publicized the spectre of over-population in his book 'Principles of Population' (1978) and claimed that population increase occurred geometrically while agricultural output could only be raised arithmetically.[23]

The race between food production and growth of population is too clear. The existing and impending crises in human nutrition and living conditions are well-documented but not widely understood. As a result of improved methods of surveillance and control of disease, particularly communicable, and changes in environment, the country is caught up in the vortex of population explosion, one of the most ecological factors that has the capacity to lead to the so called 'ecocatastrophes' if not checked promptly.[24] In India, by the year 2000 A.D. at the existing level of population growth rates, the food production will have to be doubled just to maintain the same levels of inadequate nutrition as of today and tribled if nutrition is to be brought upto the minimum requirements as recommended by nutrition experts.[25]

Population growth, poor nutrition, high infant and child mortality and low incomes form a vicious circle. Mortality among infants and toddlers is high largely due to the high prevalence of mal-nutrition and associated childhood infections. One of the causes attributed to the failure of family planning is that mal-nutrition contributes to a high death rate among the children and that this in turn acts as a disincentive for the parents to limit the number of births in family. If this general experience of losing children were to change for the better, many more parents might be willing to limit their family.

Increasing population pressure also brings about re-distribution and migration of population from rural to urban areas. One of the phenomena that occurs during such a process of urbanization is changes in the dietary practices like preferring bottle feeding to breast milk etc. In fact, surveys carried out revealed that the nutritional status of the urban poor (slum dwellers) is worse than their rural counterparts.

Population Density

A study of the density of population per sq. km. gives some clues to the understanding of the state of health of the people. More closely populated areas usually have adverse man-land ratio and hence poorer standard of living which in turn lead to poor health. This is especially the case in a country like India where a great majority of the people depend on agriculture for their livelihood. Densely populated areas have poorer sanitation and people living there are more susceptible to epidemic and other diseases than others.

The mean density of population in the area (2001) was 820 persons per sq. km. A very heavy concentration of population is found in the belt consisting of the irrigated Ganga Plains. More than a half of the country's population is concentrated in one-fifth of its area. In contrast to the plains of the country, peninsular India in general has relatively low density of population. However, many persons live in relation to the available land resources in the middle and lower Ganga Valley. About 25 per cent of the farmers of the country live in this area with average holding per household as low as 4.3 acres. When we compare the density of population in India with that of other countries of the world, the situation does not appear to be really bad. But when we analyse in the inter-state and inter-district differences in density, we do see some areas facing heavy population pressure. To get the real picture, it is essential to relate the density to land capability, which gives the degree of over-populated or under-populated, is to be calculated on the basis of land capability.[26] Non-irrigated rice producing areas of the country are extremely over-populated. This includes east Uttar Pradesh (though whole of Uttar Pradesh itself has the population density of +700 persons per sq. km. whereas in east Uttar Pradesh, e.g. the districts of Faizabad and Sultanpur, together has the density of 820. Here the population density is more than what the land can support.

A study of pressure of population on land gives us clues to the degree of under and mal-nutrition which exists. The areas which are over-populated are likely to have food scarcities atleast at local levels, and hence are likely to suffer from under-nutrition. Geographic conditions influence the economic and social development of the people by the abundance, paucity or general character of the natural resources, by the local case or difficulty of securing the necessaries of life,[27] as by the possibility of industry, commerce, agriculture afforded by the environment.

Income Levels

Poverty is still a major problem of our masses. Nearly one-third of the total population live below the poverty line. A great majority of infant deaths takes place in families having a low income and hence low standard of living. The economic status of the parents determines the diet, housing, sanitation, medical attention and general care that the child gets. Whether these people live in rural or urban makes little difference. The incidence of mortality is always higher in lower strata than the higher class residential areas. Sydenstricker has rightly said that 'it is difficult to escape the conclusion that the major determinant in the mortality of infants over one month of age is a complex of environmental conditions among which the economic status of the family is a dominant factor'.[28] As per the census 2001, a great majority of the people in India are engaged in agriculture. They practice subsistence farming and lead a very precarious life. The income of such people is not assured, and frequent occurrence of famines and floods have almost broken the economic backbone. The average income per head of the agricultural people is as low as Rs. 4270 per annum and their expenditure per head on all necessities of life is scarcely more than 24 rupees per day. Conditions are steadily improving no doubt, but the gap between that and what ought to be is still so wide that it will take several decades before the low income people in India will be able to afford to have real good food, clothing, shelter and lead a happy life. The poorest will not be able to buy for themselves with their earnings all the essentials for a minimum standard of living; their complete earnings are spent on food alone, and still they are not able to get the required nutrients, with a per capita income of about 3278 rupees per annum it is not possible to provide enough food, what to say about nutritious food. In view of the very low purchasing power, bulk of our population depends solely on cereals and negligible amount of pulses for their calories and protein needs. Studies revealed that as the income levels go up, consumption of quality foods like milk, vegetable and fruits goes up and dependence on cereals is reduced. At the existing level of per capita incomes, we need all the land available to produce grains simply for minimal calorie intake. The income should at least rise to eight to tenfold—which at current rates of growth may take nearly a century—if one were to include reasonable amount of animal foods in the diet.

In many cases, the ailment of the infant has a relationship with the health and diet of the mother. Poor families are unable to feed the infants properly, as they are unable to generate enough milk and secondly, they often left their children half fed as they go out for work. There are cases where infants at the early age are given cereals meant for adults. This results in bloated bellies and anaemic looks—it is the common sight in our rural parts.

Beri-Beri is the disease which mostly affects the poorer, who for one reason or other, cannot afford variety foods which would balance the lack of vitamin in the rice that they consume daily. Next important disease associated mainly with poverty is Anaemia that wherever poverty and mal-nutrition exist, and an insanitary environment increases risk. Infections and infestations, absorption defects of the bowel, the character and composition of the diet itself, the place of growth and the nutritional need of an individual, the customs as marriage and child birth; and the foods permitted to pregnant and lactating women, are all immediately involved. Severe anaemia adversely affects the working capacity of the rural population and a country's economic loss due to this form of mal-nutrition is probably very great.

Agriculture, food and nutrition are inter-linked. Since independence, India has witnessed revolutionary changes in the industrial, agricultural and health spheres. Several major policies have been formulated and new strategies applied on the food and agriculture front. As a part of the Green Revolution in Indian agriculture, much attention is devoted to intensive and extensive cultivation of food grains. In this effort, it is important that all factors which can adversely affect the total yield of foodgrains are to be kept under control. While increasing total food production is important, proper selection of foods is another important aspect. When one is keen on obtaining maximum nutritional benefit from any foodstuff, its nutritional value should be known first. The pattern of agriculture activities in any community is dynamic, that is, agricultural activities are constantly adjusting to the environment, whether the environmental changes are physical, economic, political or cultural. Changes in the use of agricultural lands are part of the overall adjustment and vary considerably in time and place. Changes in the crop land use have been made with a view to introducing multiple cropping systems appropriate to each region, to intensify the introduction of relay cropping, inter-cropping and multiple cropping systems. These measures have dual advantages of improving soil fertility through introduction of a legume crop in the cycle and also improving the nutritional level of the population of the region through diversification of diets and increased availability of millets, pulses and oilseeds and also to give increased income to the farmer per unit area of land. Nutritional dimension in higher yielding varieties has been adequately cared, crops screened for their nutrients composition. High yielding varieties with higher protein, high lysine, high B-carotene, high iron in cereals and millets have been identified.

Food Consumption Pattern and Varying Food Habits

Food is the urgent and recurrent need of an individual. It dictates his activities in relation to his land at every stage of economic development, fix in the locality of the encomponent or village and determines the size of the territory from which sustenance is drawn. The length of residence in one place depends upon whether the springs of its food supply are perennial or intermittent, while the abundance of their flow determines how large a population a given piece of land can support.[29] Food shortage in India means millions of children may die before attaining the age of eight or nine months. Even with a normal harvest, nearly half the Indians live on less than 1600 calories per day and consequently a partial crop failure reduces the diet of many poor persons to disastrously low levels.[30] Besides, the overall quantity of food (wheat, rice, and other cereals), the total calories, it is essential to think of quality and quantity of proteins, one of the most serious health problem today the countries are facing, what the nutritionists call protein-calorie mal-nutrition. It is estimated that every year millions of children die and many more are retarded physically and mentally, because of inadequate protein. The mal-nourished retarded survivors will be major handicaps to the future social and economic development of the country.

Food habits of the people vary from culture to culture. It has been seen that usually people living in isolated rural community use only those, but not all, foods which are locally produced. What people are willing to eat is determined by a complex system of attitudes, ideas and assumption that form the local culture, including religious restriction, taboos and ideas pertaining to the merits and demerits of food and past practices. Food habits are, therefore, the product of the people's present environment and past history. These two factors also determine the meal pattern and methods of eating.

In India, food habits are not desirable scientific. Firstly, for a great majority of our people, food is only a means to fill the belly; in such conditions one cannot even think in terms of nutrition. It is difficult for the people to pay for a wholesome meal. Secondly, even those who can afford it, do not do so. They use items of food which is considered to be prestigious e.g. people consume polished rice because it looks better, although gives them beri-beri. Thirdly, the method of cooking is so unscientific that most of the nutrients are wasted before it is eaten. Finally, there are certain restrictions (religious, socio-cultural) which inhabit people from taking certain food items. In many families only vegetarian meals are allowed, other families make distinction between pork and other meat, or beaf and other meat. As a result, it has been seen that a large number of people suffer from mal-nutritional deficiency diseases as well as from mal or under-nutrition. Food eaten in India differs from area to area, and the diets are generally deficient in vitamin-A, suitable proteins and certain salts (Fig. 4.1).

Rice is the most important grain in the diet of more than half of the human race, especially in the wet parts of the world. In India rice constitutes the main diet of the people in Andhra Pradesh, Bihar, Himachal Pradesh, Jammu and Kashmir, Kerala, Tamil Nadu, Maharahstra, Mysore, Uttar Pradesh and West Bengal.[31] Among village people of Uttar Pradesh it is taken unpolished, known as red rice, but it is usually treated so as to lose a large part of its germ. The loss results form pounding of the kernels in rude mortars. The brainlayer, which is richer in mineral salts and the endosperm of the seed is related in this process. McCairison (1923) concluded that vitamin-A is present

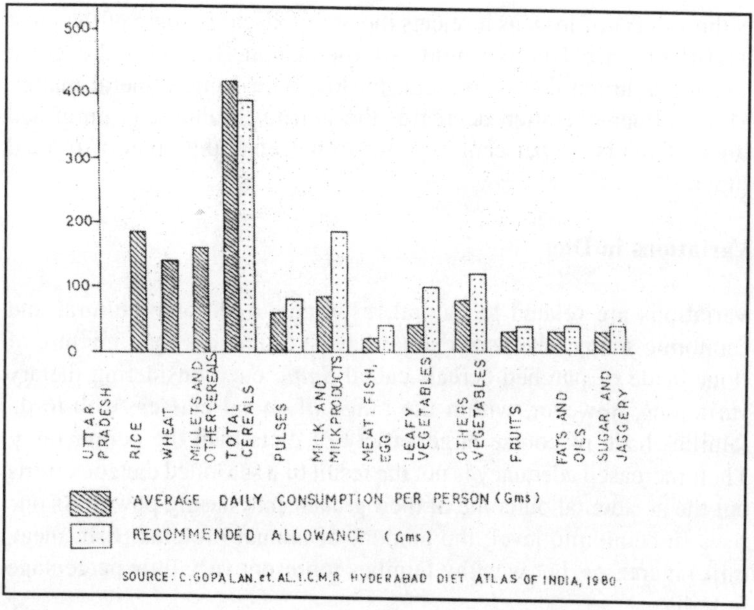

Fig. 4.1 : Uttar Pradesh Consumption Pattern of Different Food Stuffs

in paddy before it is milled.[32] According to Dr. Ansari, of all cereals, rice is the richest in starch, of which it has nearly 50 per cent, the starch in rice has further advantage of being present in small and easily digestible grains. If boiled in excess of water and it is thrown away, it will deprive of water soluable vitamin-B. In the process of polishing, all outer coverings of the grain are removed consisting of the husk as well as the pigmented covering containing vitamin-B, fat and protein necessary for health and growth. It has been proved that the absence of vitamin-B from the polished rice has been instrumental in causing beri-beri. The unpolished rice, per boiled, hand pounded, is superior to the unpolished rice turned from mills.[33]

Next to rice, comes the wheat, second most important of cereals foods in India. Although, it constitutes main diet only in the states of Madhya Pradesh, Punjab, Haryana, Rajasthan and Western Uttar Pradesh. Wheat grain consists of brain or outer envelop, mainly composed of cellulose, the Kernal consisting of starch and the germ consisting of soluable starch, protein and some fat. But again milling is the subject of loss, as it rejects the brain, discards some of the most useful chemical constituents of the wheat, for with the germ considerable amount of protein, fat lost with some mineral matter. More refinement often decreases the nutritive value, e.g. unrefined sugar (Gur) is 33 per cent superior in nutrients than that of refined sugar.

Variations in Diet

Variations are related to natural resources, traditional cultural and economic status. The poor classes have a foundness for a mixture of flour made of parched cereals called *Sattu*, etc. considering dietary variations, however, within the range of social classes, well-to-do families have of course large variety of diets than the poorer ones. Their increased adequacy is not the result of a seasoned dietetic efforts but the accidental outcome of their greater purchasing power. As one rises in economic level, the amount of annual proteins (fish, meat, milk) increases, but wealthy families represent very little percentage in India.

Nutrition and Palatability

This two situation in which food may lead to inferior nutrition—the avoidance of existing foods and the poor acceptability of new foods are well recognized. With the release of economic pressure, and in the absence of social pressure people tend to eat diets with increasing amount of animal foods. This implies that these protein-rich foods are more palatable than the strach rich vegetable foods, our preference for the animal foods, their high palatability is good in its nutritional value. But this is not universal. There are exceptions in both directions. There existing foods of low palatability but of high nutritional value, and conversely foods of high palatability but of low or even undesirable value. The same attitude accounts for the view that sugar is good, especially for children, because they like sweets. This is the most important example of the disassociation between palatability and nutrition, and are of the main reasons why the nutritional studies are so connected with the changing food habits.

Social, economic and geographical factors determine the diet of a region. The faults determine the types of diseases, e.g. Pellagra is associated with diets lacking nicotinic acid, beri-beri is associated with rice eating population and so on.

The roots of our environmental troubles are largely religious, according to Lynn White J.R., the attitudes and actions of modern technological man contradict the reality that the man is part of nature, not rightful master over nature.[34] Religious and social customs not only hinder agricultural development, but also restrict the population in their dieting habits. In Indonesia, milk is not given to children because it is considered unhealthy for them. In Malaysia, children are doubly handicapped, they are not given fish and meat as they are supposed to give them worms. It is tempting to suppose that many of the customs which restrict the consumption of foods, mostly of the protein—rich and more expensive food e.g. meat, eggs, milk had their origin in economics. However, it is interesting to note that restrictions are mostly on mothers and children who need it more than man.[35] Among Muslims, however, women are restricted to rice only, for forty days after the birth of a child, besides the distinctions between vegetarian and non-vegetarian and the diets prescribed for different physiological conditions. As a result, we find a large number of deficiency diseases arising to these factors. These factors also affect directly the infant mortality.

C. *Biological Environment*

Another approach to the study of the geographical distribution of diseases could be based on the relationships between certain diseases and certain diets. The diseases could be, of course, caused by parasitic infection, by the nature of the food ingested, or both such as milk and fish.

Rice is the food consumed by the majority in India, in certain regions together with other foods. The diseases associated with rice can be classified in two groups : firstly, related to cultivation and secondly, those related to consumption. The prevalence of malaria is closely associated with the cultivation of rice. Although this statement is true in general, it is qualified by the fact that each region has its own malaria vector and each vector has its own living habits. The vector which breeds in the stagnating water of the field, is a weak carrier, and it has, therefore, been though possible to combat malaria in the islands by developing rice culture.

Many other diseases directly related to the intake of food result from (i) food-borne intoxication or (ii) food-borne infection. In the latter category some diseases like salmonellas including typhoid fever, diphtheria, shigellosis, amoebiasis, tuberculosis, brucellosis scarlet fever, helminithiasis, etc.

Water Supply

Water for drinking or for domestic use influences the public health. Some diseases are water-borne, directly or indirectly. This being the importance of water for survival, man has tried from time immemorial to have a dependable clean water supply. Earlier people believed that 'it is good to keep water in copper vessels, to expose to sunlight and filter through charcoal'.[36] Today not more than 25 per cent of urban centres and 10 per cent of the rural settlements have the benefit of protected water supply.

Man gets drinking water from various sources, e.g. from water pumps, wells, springs, rivers, lakes, ponds and rains. Related to each of these sources are factors producing or inhabiting disease. Lack of iodine in water causes foiler, the fluorine content of water governs several pathological conditions. If its content is lower than one part per million, dental carries is common; if much higher, neoetted enamel (dental flourosis) occurs. Calcium deficiency in water may result in the causation of rickets and osteomalacia or at least combines with other factors to produce them. Excess of it with phosphate disturb gastro-intestinal setup and facilitates the production of stones. Calcium deficiency not only exists in water but also in the vegetable grown. There are a number of other disease which can be caused due to sewage pollution in water supply. Wells in the villages are rarely covered and hence leaves and dust have unhindered entry into them. When the leaves rot in water, they not only create a foul smell but also give rise to organisms which, when swallowed with water by men or animals, give rise to several diseases.

It has been realised that environmental sanitation contribute much to environmental health. In ancient period the basis of their civilization was the sanitary installations. The need for a healthful environment is common to all people; it cuts across boundaries of occupations, races, classes and politics. It differs from neighbourhood to neighbourhood and from region to region, not in fundamental but in complexity.[37] It is difficult to improve the whole country at the certain level of standard by propagating environmental health awareness throughout the communities. The agriculturists in the rural areas of the west are facing somewhat different problems in comparison to the agriculturists in the rural areas of the east. Such regional variations in environmental conditions have been observed in other communities of the country. These variations lead to different types of environmental diseases, deficiency as well as communicable.[38]

House and city planning also exerts its effect on the community health. We have to think much of disease than of health, from this view point all the factors which affect health, housing problems come to fore-front. As the slum of the day is no longer a lot bed of cholera but it will remain, however, a major source of pollution of physical environment. The dwellers in poor housing are subjected to many-fold problems, i.e. low income, mal-nourishment, limited education. In due course of time, these complex problems beget ill health among the dwellers in the poor housing areas. The sun-shine must reach the skin, and its avoidance encourages rickets and osteomalacia among the dwellers. The high incidence of rickets is found in the Kangara valley of Punjab, due to combination of high population pressure on the cultivated land, itself poor in lime and phosphorus and diet excessively cereal based with improper housing.

Deficiency Diseases

Human beings are involved in many economic activities to gain a livelihood, but none of these activities are so fundamental to this existence as agriculture because it provides sustenance to nearly 85 per cent of the total population in the area. Consciously used, the natural environment provides habitat for their crops and animals.

Here the natural environment is the 'Land', which is the basic resource of the farmers. The inherent qualities of the land, the growing population pressure, the degree of socio-cultural advancement are important factors, restricting farmer's choice and response. Any crop which is produced in the field requires labour and capital inputs in varying proportions and intensities and the output is consumed by the rural community as well as the non-agriculturist.

The forms of agricultural activities found in any region are response to four groups of environmental factors: (i) Physical, (ii) Socio-cultural, (iii) Economic and (iv) Political.

The physical factors relate to climate, geomorphology, vegetation and soil which combine to provide the ecological limits within which particular crops may be grown on a profitable basis. They provide essential nutrients and minerals which are important for human beings, e.g. iodine but unfortunately it is deficient in the area under study.

The socio-cultural factors are related to the activities of the people through ages, and may condition acceptance of change in agricultural and dietary habits. They also include religion and social organizations which impinge upon farming activities and group the entire population into vegetarian and non-vegetarian categories. They very often put certain restrictions under which one community can take certain items of food while the other cannot. Different communities observe different cultures, e.g. Muslim women after delivery remains confined to their houses for about forty days while the other communities do not follow such restrictions.

Economic factors are related to the relative profitability of the crops produced, its availability, distribution among the rural community, purchasing power of the farmers to buy modern machinery/fertilizers, water for irrigation and new varieties of seed etc. For the improvement of their agriculture and also to buy from the market if necessary, enough food to enable them to maintain sound health. Political factors very often play important role in so far as the availability, distribution, price support or crops subsidies have to be decided by the district officials dealing with such problems.

Further political factors are related to the government plans, decisions aimed at assisting or retarding agricultural development and measures in respect of community health programmes, e.g. direct subsidy, acreage limitations, provision of scientific research in agricultural development and health awareness programmes, family planning and programmes relating to dietary habits and health.

In the developing countries like ours where farming techniques are not mechanized and system relating to exchange of commodities is not well-developed, physical and socio-cultural factors generally determine the agricultural activities. The success of this system depends on a balance between the two, i.e. energy input and production of food stuff or energy output. As the farmer clears the land, cultivates the soil, sows seeds and weeds the crops, he is providing inputs of energy for the system, which operates through the medium of land; also the system is getting inputs of energy through natural resources, i.e. sun-shine, rainfall, which also operates through the medium of land. The combined energy inputs result in an energy output from the land in the form of food, which gives human being the essential nutrient required to avoid deficiency diseases and to maintain normal health. So the output must be equal to man's energy inputs plus conversion losses if the system is to be self-perpetuating. There may be appreciable loss of energy in religious, social and ceremonial activities, and clearing weeds or secondary wild growth which are important competitors of the food crops and other such agricultural and non-agricultural activities. Nor do all natural energy result in food growth, i.e. weeds and secondary wild growth. The food stuff thus produced, if not enough to satisfy the hunger or equal to the inputs, the system cannot continue its cycle successfully.

Assuming natural energy input (constant) in any locality, man's ability to drive sufficient energy from the land depends upon two factors: his own energy inputs and ability of land to convert the supplies of energy to food stuff, which will vary directly with fertility factors and agricultural techniques. Reduction in soil fertility decrease the efficiency of man's energy inputs with constant higher energy losses and reduced supply of energy to man via food supply (Fig. 4.2). Reduced supply of food will result in reduced conversion to exchange value reduced capital input and reduced supply of essential food elements, i.e. protein, fat, carbohydrates, calcium, iron, vitamins and

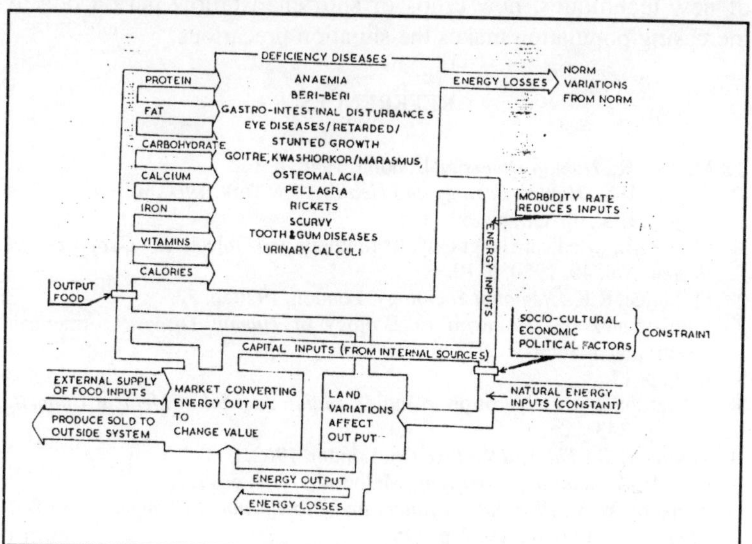

Fig. 4.2 : Correlation between deficiency deseases and environment of factors

calories, which are essential for a normal health. Naturally the reduced output of food elements results in increased morbidity rate and exposed the rural community to different nutritional deficiency diseases, like Anaemia, Beri-Beri and gastro nutritional disturbances, eye diseases, and related diseases, goitre, kwashiorkor/marasmus, osteomalacia, pellagra, rickets, scurvy/tooth and gum and urinary culculi. Increased morbidity rate reduces the input of energy because a sick man cannot perform equal to healthy man. Further, more environmental factors discussed earlier may be termed as bottleneck, reduces the flow of energy input to the land and these variations ultimately affect the outputs. The environmental factors which are affecting agricultural production are also responsible for the farmers health as whatever food stuff is available to the farming community and obtained from the market through exchange are not equally distributed and the community cannot eat what they have to eat. Thus an agricultural labour is not having the privileges which a farm owner has or what one sect is eating another cannot; that makes the situation more worst. The constant energy inputs may not be the same variation is total energy input may be allowed. Man is trying to grow as much as possible to maintain balance by adopting all the possible inputs, e.g. adoption of new techniques, new crops or shortened fallow period due to increasing population makes the situation precarious.

REFERENCES

1. Mathur, K., *Human Diversity*, London, 1946, p. 11.
2. Rogers, E.S., *Human Ecology and Health*, New York, 1960, p. 167.
3. Rogers, E.S., op. cit., p. 169.
4. May, J.M., 'Medical Geography, Its Methods and Objectives', *Geographical Review*, Vol. 40, 1950, p. 10.
5. Mukerjee, R.K., *Regional Sociology*, London, 1926, p. 32.
6. Marti-Ibanez, F., *Foreword to Ecology of Human Diseases*, American Geographical Society, 1958, p. 17.
7. *Ibid.*, p. 17.
8. Patwardhan, V.N. 'Nutrition in India', *Indian Journal of Medical Council*, 1962, p. 343.
9. Moore, W.G., *The Soil We Live On*, London 1962, p. 3.
10. Lant, P., *Agriculture Geography*, Melborne, 1968, p. 77.
11. Albrecht, W.A., *Physical, Chemical and Bio-Chemical Changes in the Soil Community*, London, 1967, p. 395.
12. F.A.O., 'Conflicting Doctrines about Soils' Reprint from the *Scientific Monthly*, Vol. LXXI, No. 6, Washington, June 1948, pp. 7-16.
13. Diell, S.H., *Healthful Living*, New York 1964, p. 445.

14. Huntington, E., *Main Springs of Civilization*, New York, 1945.
15. Markham, S. F., *Climate and the Energy of Nations*, London, 1942, p. 112.
16. Klages Karl, H.W., *Ecological Crop Geography* New York, 1954, p. 47.
17. U.S. Department of Agriculture: *Climate and Man*, Washington, D.C., 1941, p. 256.
18. Lee, D.H.K., 'Physiology and Tropics', *Malayan Medieval Journal*, 1930, p. 105.
19. Lee, D.H.K., *Climate and Economic Development in the Tropics*, Singapore, p. 106.
20. Amar, H., *The Sociological Approach to Problems of Community Development*, Arab States Fundamental Education Centre, Sirs-et-Layyan, U.A.R., 1960, p.36.
21. Rehman, J., *Health and Environment,* T.C.M., Aligarh, 1968, p. 17.
22. Detwyler, T.R., *Man's Impact on Environment*, New York, 1921, p. 36.
23. Morgan, W.B. and Munton, R.J.C., *Agriculture Geography*, London, 1971, p. 58.
24. Vijayaraghvan, K., *Ecological Constraints and Nutritional Status of the Community*, Nutrition – C.U.R., Hyderabad, July, 1974, p. 14.
25. Vijayaraghvan, K., op. cit., p. 14.
26. Gupta, P.S. and Solasyuk, G., *Economic Rationalization of India: Problems and Approach*, Census of India, New Delhi, 1981.
27. Sample, E.C., *Influence of Geographic Environment*, London, 1911, p. 43.
28. Sydenstricker, E., *Health and Environment*, New York, 1937, p. 84.
29. Sample, E.C., *op. cit*., p. 61.
30. Wilson, B.R., *Environmental Problems*, U.S.A., 1968, p. 18.
31. *Diet Atlas of India*, Hyderabad, 1987, pp. 25-29.
32. Gandhi, M.K., *Diet and Diet Reform*, Ahmadabad, 1949, p. 43.
33. *Ibid.*, p.44
34. Detwyler, T.R., *op. cit*., p. 27
35. Yukdin, J. and Makenzie, T.C. (Edited), *Charging Food Habits*, London, 1964, p. 16.
36. Kawata, K., *Environmental Sanitation in India*, Ludhiana, 1963, pp. 9-10.
37. *Ibid.*
38. Ahmad, S.W., *Distribution of Nutritional Deficiency Disease in Relation to Environmental Factors in Central Ganga-Ghaghra Doab,* Aligarh, 1975, p. 43.

5 Case study of the selected villages

(A micro level study)

Methodology and Collection of Data

While selecting the villages for detailed study of various deficiency diseases, the author has visited large number of villages of the area under study, taking into consideration the time constraints and the total funds available, the author has surveyed twelve villages for the present project. Many of these villages, as it has been observed, show a concentration of the various deficiency diseases. Since the study area lies in a homogenous plain with little variations in the topographical features, agricultural practices, types of crops produced, level of economic status, dietary habits and environmental conditions, it has become almost an easy task for the researcher to select villages adopting the technique of purposive sampling. Under the existing conditions the present technique will not lead to any kind of generalization of result, rather it is bound to convey the real position with regard to the existence of various deficiency diseases with which the rural communities are confronting. It is possible that one may come across such instances where variations in the occurrence of various deficiency diseases are located for which the author has been attracted to study. Some villages may exhibit mostly all the diseases while others may have only a few, the author has noticed that there are certain villages where the number of such diseases is relatively small in agricultural prosperous villages. These villages have better literacy, irrigation facilities and also having better Socio-economic environment. The other category of villages having meagre facilities relating to irrigation water, fertilizers, literacy and sources of income exhibit larger number of such diseases. Such villages may be classed as agriculturally backward. After selecting the villages the author is to adopt a methodology which may ensure a satisfactory conduct of deficiency disease survey. For this purpose, the total population of the selected villages have been classified in three economic groups i.e. A.B.C. and detailed dietary and disease survey in these three economic groups, of people was conducted with a view to assess their nutritional status. Such groups have been made after assessing their total income from all sources. This income stratification gives a clear indication of the economic status of the village community. The stratification as suggested by the author is based on the actual survey of the villages under study and may be stated as under :

A. Group/category (Above Rs. 1500 per head per month)
B. Group/category (Rs. 800-1500 per head per month)
C. Group/category (Below Rs. 800 per head per month)

This survey is spread over in three climatic seasons and covering two agricultural seasons of the year as the villagers depend for their daily food on the crops produced during these periods and to assess the effect of seasonal variations in food intake and daily availability of nutrition from the food and other eatables and drinks. The village communities were asked to recall all the foods they had consumed on the previous day and the frequency of consumption of various foods during the last week and the entire month. The survey was conducted for a month in each season, without prior information to the rural community, so that any cautious deviation from the rural daily intake could be avoided. The information so gathered had been processed and a dietary intake sheet was prepared. This helped in getting information regarding calories intake together with other important nutrients in their diets. Further, it was found that, in general, people suffered from under and mal-nutrition both.

Regarding the prevalence of deficiency diseases, the patients in the selected villages with developed and semi-developed symptoms were interviewed during the door to door survey and discussed the problem at length with local doctor's checked their records and the records of state government hospitals as well in respect of these diseases.

Before taking up individual villages for a detailed study of nutritional deficiency disease, it will be worthwhile to consider the food items available to the rural population from within and as well as from outside the villages under study. There are two main crop seasons, i.e. kharif and rabi. In the kharif season, rice millets (small and large), maize are the main crops while in the rabi season, wheat, barley, gram, peas, arhar (pulses) and groundnuts are cultivated. Besides these many pulses (locally known as Moong Urd, Masoor, etc.), oilseeds, linseed, potatoes and sugarcane are also grown. These crops form the basic items of food for the rural population. The entire caloric intake derived from these sources except in some villages where the population is economically well off, and can afford to purchase some fruits and other nutritive items of food.

On the whole, the major sources of daily foods in the rural areas are agriculture. If the agricultural returns are good, their economic condition will be better and they are excepted to have better diet, and health. In the under developed villages, on account of poor diets, people have ill-health. Besides these, some other important environmental factors have to be considered.

Birth

Customs relating to birth are simple in all castes and communities but not good for health. When women conceive, there is no proper care about her diet and health. She has to live on ordinary diets throughout the period of pregnancy. She is in most cases confined to a dark and unhygienic room where her baby is being kept. She is not provided with nutritive diets throughout this period, which a mother giving birth to a child needs. However, in some well-do-to families, some nourishing diets are given to such mother only for a week or so. In most cases she is not exposed to the sun, she is not exposed to fresh air and in most of the cases, damp, dark small mud room with smoke is considered highly unhygienic for the mother and the baby.

House Types

The structure and type of dwelling and the quality of construction material in the rural areas usually lead to unhygienic conditions. Wherein the rural communities have to pass their lives. Most of the dwellings are made of mud with tiles on the roof. These tiles are placed on bamboos or wood logs, which rest on the two ends of the walls and have downwards slope. Mud is also used for roofing in Sultanpur district. An average house has a thatched or tiled varandah, enclosed courtyard along the side of which are built one or two small rooms without proper ventilation and sometimes without it. The cattle are kept in the front enclosed varandah through which main entrance is usually found. The well-to-do families have very often separate place made of bricks and cement.

Though, the mud houses are simple and economical yet uncomfortable and unsafe during the rainy season. They very often leak when torrential rain occurs and unsanitary conditions prevail. These houses are without urinals, latrines and bathrooms. The villagers are used to go to nearby fields to answer the call of nature. As mentioned earlier *kotheries* (small rooms) often dark without ventilation are often used for bath by the young women and girls. All the houses have to drain out filthy water into the lanes, making movement difficult. They have limited sources for improvement in their living conditions and as a result a unhygienic condition prevails throughout.

Food and Drinks

There is not much difference in the pattern of food consumption; majority of the people eat course grains. They take pulses or vegetables with the principal meals. Sometimes they take only one food stuff (peas or grams) in both the diets. The use of wheat flour is either confined to upper strata and to some extent middle strata and that too on festivals. Rice is the staple item of the diet; vegetables are generally produced locally and are available on market days. Non-vegetarian foods are not consumed regularly even by the non-vegetarian but like vegetable, weekly market provides non-vegetarian items.

Milk and ghee are generally costly items and are not affordable to the majority of rural popoulation due to economic reasons. The villagers eat melons, water melons, cheap variety of mango, mahua, during summer and rainy season as supplementary diet. Sweets are prepared occasionally. The use of refined sugar is rare but *gur* (raw sugar) is largely consumed. Tea consumption is confined to a small section, though in winters, its use increases. Smoking is a special feature of the rural community and some of them also use betal leaves and country made liquor. Out of the total house holds surveyed, only 25 per cent take food three times a day, 68 per cent two times and 7 per cent one time a day. The frequency of meals depends on the economic status of the household. The absence or lack of milk, ghee, animal food and vegetable makes the daily diets sub-nutritious. The intake of calcium, protein, fat, vitamin-A, C and other nutrients are not satisfactory. So in the absence of protective foods, better health conditions cannot be expected and people are highly-prone to various diseases, particularly deficiency diseases like anaemia, beri-beri and gastro intestinal, disturbances, scurvy, tooth and gum diseases, rickets, goitre, eye diseases, retarded growth, kwashiorker, marasmus, osteomalacia, diabetes etc.

Mumtaz Nagar

The village Mumtaz Nagar lies at a distance of 7 km from Faizabad town on the bank of river Ghaghra at 26° 47″ north latitude and 82°04′56″ east longitude. The district has two categories of soil, viz. the khadar and the bhangar. Though it has two soil groups, khadar soil occurs, in the immediate neighborhood of the river Ghaghra and bhangar soil is found across the road on higher lands. Bhangar is devoted to double cropping and gives higher returns per acre whereas khadar is mainly devoted to one crop either cereal or pulses but often put to zaid cash crops too, e.g. melons, water melons etc. Vegetables including potatoes are also cultivated in the village but on a very small and large scale depending on the size of the individual holdings of the farmers.

The population of the village in 2001 was 1260 consisting of 557 males, 462 females and 241 children. It is not purely a vegetarian village. About 40 per cent of the residents are non-vegetarian under A, B and C categories,[1] but the supply of the essential nutrients are inadequate in both the groups in the above said categories, with the caloric intake of 1968 in category C to 2503 in category A per head per day. The main sources of calories are cereals but about 80 per cent of the population does not get the standard requirement of 2400 calories from all sources per head per day, with the result that about 14.2 per cent of the rural population is liable to various deficiency diseases. The most common among the deficiency diseases is goitre, which claims the higher percentage of about 13.5 per cent. Although goitre is not a killing disease, yet it creates problems for the patients, who feel physically inactive. This is of Terai origin and often found in the khadar areas. On the whole, death due to the deficiency diseases found among the villagers accounted for about 2.7 per cent of the total deaths in this village during the year 2001.

It is clear from Table 5.1 that the nutritional positions of the inhabitants is not satisfactory and people are exposed to various deficiency diseases. Moreover, the supply of various nutrients are not

Table 5.1 : Mumtaz Nagar : Supply of Different Nutrients per head per day in the Categories A, B, C, and percentage of Departure from Standard Requirement

Elements of Food	*Standard Requirement*	*Actual Intake* A	*Actual Intake* B	*Actual Intake* C	*PDSR* A	*PDSR* B	*PDSR* C
Protein g	68	66.6	46.9	32.0	-2.1	-31.0	-52.9
Fat g	50	36.9	22.2	11.8	-26.2	-55.6	-76.4
Carbohydrate g	440	450.6	460.8	472.9	+2.4	+4.7	+7.5
Calcium mg	700	544.3	481.5	287.5	-22.2	-31.2	-58.9
Iron mg	22.5	53.8	59.9	47.9	+138.8	+166.3	+112.8
Vitamin-A I.U.	3500	2809	1049	1024.6	-19.7	-70.0	-70.7
Thiamine mg	1.12	2.0	2.1	2.2	+78.5	+87.5	+93.8
Riboflavin mg	1.46	2.2	1.05	1.2	+57.7	-28.1	-17.8
Niacin mg	19	24.6	19.6	15.6	+29.4	+3.1	-17.9
Vitamin-C mg	43	17.3	15.0	13.9	-59.8	-65.1	-67.6
Calories	2400	2503	1931	1968.6	+4.2	-19.5	-29.2

PDSR — Refers to percentage of departure from standard requirement.
— Deficiency
— Surplus
Source : Based on field survey conducted in 2001.

uniform in all these categories, viz. the supply of iron, carbohydrate, thiamine and to some extent protein and niacin is fairly high in all the three categories in comparison to the supply of fat, calcium, vitamin-A and C which are deficient to the tune of –26.2, –22.2, –19.7 and –59.8 per cent respectively among the people of category A, while in the case of categories B and C, they are deficient to the level of –55.6, –31.2, –70.0, –65.1 per cent and –76.4, –58.9, –70.7, –67.6 per cent respectively per head per day. The supply of riboflavin is also short by –28.1 per cent in case of B category, riboflavin along with niacin are deficient in category C, by –17.8 and –17.9 per cent. Whereas these two nutrients were fairly supplied among the families of category A.

The supply of iodine though uniform among the different categories is deficient and has created many health problems. Deficiency of iodine in water available for drinking has been observed and no alternative arrangement to make up the deficiency is possible.

Table 5.1 have been prepared on the basis of data collected by the author regarding the diets of the villagers in three different seasons. The table shows the per head per day intake of calories and other essential nutrients of food, together with the standard requirement and their percentage of departure from the standard requirement.[2]

Out of the total population of 1260 about 19.6 per cent are sick, among which 65.7 per cent are deficiency patients and majority is from C category. Goitre,[3] Scurvy[4] together with tooth and gum diseases and Beri-Beri[5] accounted for the large percentage of the patients. Due to acute deficiency of iodine about 13.5 per cent of the total patients suffered from goitre alone while scurvy, tooth and gum diseases and beri-beri account for 13.7 per cent and 15.6 per cent respectively. Vitamin-A deficiency claims 11.7 per cent out of the total deficiency patients, leading to night blindness[6], kerotomalacia[7], Xerophthalmia.[8]

Deficiency of thiamine, riboflavin and niacin helps in promoting conditions for gastro-intestinal disorder, colitis, pellagra. Thiamine is not deficient but deficiencies of other nutrients may check the proper absorption of this nutrient. The shortage of riboflavin, niacin and vitamin-C together makes the situation a bit more complicated, specially among the rural communities belonging to category C. Pellagra[9] is purely a disease of lower income group, which is caused by niacin alone. This disease accounted for 3.7 per cent of the total deficiency patients in the village. Combined deficiency also causes mascular wasting and enlargement of heart in severe cases.

Vitamin-D is also scanty with the result that some of them are prone to specific disease caused due to deficient supply or availability of vitamin-D to an individual. Its deficiency also checks the absorption of phosphorus. The disease associated with this is known as 'Rickets'[10], and accounts for 14.2 per cent of death. Best way to get this vitamin is through the sun. It is more prevalent among children and women, who are generally confined within four walls of their houses.[11]

The supply of iron is in surplus almost in every category, but due to non-absorption of iron in the body or loss of blood on account of injuries etc., anemic conditions result, particularly among women and children. Açcording to Srikantia (1975), pre-school children and women in the reproductive age are the worst sufferers of anaemia. A sample survey conducted on all India, reveals that 40 per cent of the children and every second women in the country suffered from the disability, resulting in morbidity, illness and mortality.[12] Further, iron deficiency in the body is mainly responsible for this, though iron is adequately present in the diet, it is not absorbed due to various reasons.

Protein supply is a worldwide problem and is more acute in developing countries, where the average income is low and very low. Level of protein supply in the village is also not satisfactory; it is short supplied by –2.1, –31.0, –52.9 per cent in the A, B, C, categories respectively. It is clear from the given table that the deficiency is more severe in the case of category C. Naturally the highest percentage of patients suffering from Kwashiorkor[13] is from lower income group which accounts for 5.5 per cent of the total deficiency patients. What is required for a good diet is not just any Protein, but one that is well-balanced in amino-acids and has a higher biological value and protein efficiency ratio.[14] Kwashiorkor is found in Africa, India, Indonesia, Central and South America, Fiji Island etc.[15]

Besides these diseases, diabetes and urinary-calculi, osteomalacia are found in the village at the rate of 8.2, 1.3 and 2.4 per cent respectively. Excessive use of raw sugar (*gur*), hampers to produce insulin and results in diabetes. Urinary-calculi begins with the deficiency of fat soluble vitamins, calcium and phosphorus, while the osteomalasia spreads with the deficiency of calcium, phosphorus and vitamin-D. As discussed earlier, the supply of these elements in foods in the village community under study is far from satisfactory, and results in several deficiency diseases in the various categories but most affected people are the low income group.

Mullathi Barasin

It is a medium size village, about 15 km west of Sultanpur, connected by a unmetalled road on which private buses ply in all seasons. It becomes slushy during the rains, and is located in 26°21′37″ north latitude and 81°58′09″ east latitude. The shape of the village is an irregular triangle and is subject to changes due to soil erosion caused by occasional floods. The population of Mullathi is 669 consisting of 531 Hindus and 138 Muslims. Hindus are divided in four castes, namely *mallah*, *kayastha*, *teli* and *dhobi*, the last named being the only scheduled caste in the village. Mallah are in large numbers divided into 62 households. Muslims constitute about 20 per cent of the total population.

Mallahs are clustered in the centre, kayasthas live in the south-west, Muslims in the north, others are congregated in its eastern part. There is a grouping of houses on the caste basis. The physical features of the village are truly characterized by the Ganga Plain. It is situated on a raised surface and may be divided into two natural divisions : (a) the low lying in the east, inundated every year by the Gomti. Some land is annually eroded or transformed into sand soil is mostly *balua* (sandy) and is not good for cultivations, melons, watermelons and sweet potatoes are grown in the tract; (b) the level plane has a gradual and uniform slope from north-west to south-east. It is most fertile and devoted to wheat, gram, pulses in the rabi and paddy, maize, bajra in the kharif season.

Kayasthas being better placed own 1/5th of the total cultivated land and are well-to-do. Mallah are in good number and are mostly fishers and sailors but their second occupation is agriculture. They are good farmers and assisted well by their women folks. Most of them are not having any land and they earn their livelihood by string making or boat rowing, getting grains at the harvest from the farmers and get a little amount in cash from the passengers. Likewise *dhobi* (washerman) and other community members are also directly or indirectly dependent on the local food or thing available in weekly markets, e.g. meat, grains and vegetables etc. Number of vegetarians are estimated to be 55 per cent. Fish is used more commonly in the village than meat. There are two principal crops seasons, i.e. rabi and kharif with zaid in the sandy areas. Paddy occupies the low lying fields and upper land is given to other crops, i.e. wheat, barley, gram, a little arhar (pulses) and moong, the other small millets (kodon, sawan, kakun) but these small millets are generally sold out. Bajra, jowar, bejhar are locally consumed.

The daily intake of calories varies between 1807 and 2433 and is mainly based on the supply of cereals, pulses and vegetables. Domestic animals contribute milk to the diets of those who can afford it. Fish is easily available although meat is also consumed on weekends (market days) or after fortnight among the Muslims and non-Muslims. Fruits, like mangoes, guava, plums etc. are taken at negligible level.

The main source of nutrients in this village are the foodgrains, pulses, vegetables. Fish and meat are consumed to some extent in some families. Detailed picture of their nutritional position has been shown in Table 5.2. However, the caloric intake varies from 2,433 in case of category A to 2,163 and 1,807 per head per day in categories B and C respectively. Majority of the population is mal-nourished and in some cases under-nourished, with the result that about 13.6 per cent of the total population is liable to different deficiency diseases among the villagers. During the year 2001 about 1.9 per cent died on account of the various deficiency diseases in this village.

Table 5.2 is prepared on the basis of data collected, taking into consideration the standard requirement and their percentage of departure. Negative and a very high percentage of departure from the standard requirement is an alarming signal of deficiency diseases. There is a close relationship between the supply of nutrients and the deficiency diseases to be found in particular areas. The supply of different nutrients are not uniformly distributed among the village communities, Fat, calcium, vitamin-A and C and protein are not supplied properly. However the position with regard to the supply of calcium, vitamin-A is better in comparison to other villages. This is perhaps due to intake of fish and meat in B and C categories. Further, it is seen that there is surplus supply of iron, thiamine and fair supply of carbohydrate, riboflavin and niacin among the well-to-do families of the village. Among the last two categories, the supply of these elements are not adequate. They are deficient in calories as well. Supply of fat, calcium vitamin-A and C and protein is deficient to the tune of –49.8, –12.9, –35.1, 32.8, –15.4 per cent in category A, while in case of B and C categories, it is short to the tune of –61.5, –49.4, –20.6, –64.4, –18.7 and –76.0, –43.2, –23.9, –69.2, –45.9 per cent respectively per head per day. Some case of iodine deficiency is also reported. Out of the total patients, deficiency diseases account for

Table 5.2 : Mullathi Barasin : Supply of Different Nutrients per head per day in the Categories A, B, C, and percentage of Departure from Standard Requirement

Elements of Food	*Standard Requirement*	*Actual Intake* A	*Actual Intake* B	*Actual Intake* C	*PDSR* A	*PDSR* B	*PDSR* C
Protein g	68	57.5	55.3	36.8	-15.4	-18.7	-45.9
Fat g	50	25.1	19.6	12.0	-49.8	-61.5	-76.0
Carbohydrate g	440	485.9	479.7	440.6	+10.4	+9.0	-0.13
Calcium mg	700	609.1	354.2	397.6	-12.9	-49.4	-43.2
Iron mg	22.5	78.7	43.9	30.8	+150.1	+91.1	+36.9
Vitamin-A I.U.	3500	2271.6	2777	2663.5	-35.1	-20.6	-23.9
Thiamine mg	1.12	2.04	.98	2.03	+82.1	-12.5	+81.2
Riboflavin mg	1.46	1.84	1.69	1.3	+26.0	+15.7	-10.9
Niacin mg	19	20.0	19.7	19.4	+5.3	+3.7	+2.1
Vitamin-C mg	43	28.9	15.3	13.2	-32.8	-64.4	-69.2
Calories	2400	2433	2163	1807	+1.4	-9.9	-24.7

about 70.1 per cent and larger percentage is reported from the last two categories.

Deficiency of vitamin-A and C, riboflavin and iodine are responsible for more than 60 per cent of the deficiency patients surveyed in the village. Acute shortage of vitamin-C, in all the three categories caused severe damage to health, in the form of tooth and gum diseases and scurvy, which accounts for 19.2 per cent of the total deficiency patients, the highest among the deficiency diseases. Next comes the beri-beri and pellagra and eye diseases and anaemia. Due to short supply of iodine and riboflavin, niacin about 12.2 and 14.2 per cent of the deficiency disease patients are suffering from full to mild symptoms of beri-beri, gastro-intestinal disturbances and pellagra.

The cases of beri-beri are mostly from B and C categories where the supply of related nutrients is not satisfactory. While eye disease and anaemia accounted for 15.9 per cent and 11.9 per cent respectively and are confined usually to C category, where the supply of vitamin-A is –23.9 per cent below the standard requirement, causing eye defects i.e., night blindness, xerophthalmia and also checks the proper growth and cause dry beri-beri. Its deficiency coupled with shortage of calcium and fat caused osteomalacia, urinary calculi 2.1, 2.3 per cent respectively. Although iron is supplied fairly, yet anaemia accounts for 11.9 per cent among which more than 8.5 per cent are women and rest 3.4 per cent are children; it may be due to mal-absorption of iron in the body or due to absence of other nutrients.

Besides these deficiency diseases, rickets, kwashiorkor, marasmus and diabetes are also noticed. Deficiency of vitamin-D, protein and insulin in the body helps in promoting these deficiency diseases and the patients suffering from these diseases are 7.3, 9.7 and 5.1 per cent respectively.

Due to the short supply of vitamin-D to the village population ricket is a common disease among children of low income group. Its deficiency also checks the absorption of phosphorus. Protein supply is deficient in almost the entire village population. Due to excessive use of sugar, related metabolism failed in absorbing sugar, with the result that sugar passes directly in the blood and the patient suffers from diabetes due to lack of insulin in the body.

Dhanipur

This village lies at a distance of about 20 km west of Faizabad town in the sandy loam soil and is located in 82°58′30″ north latitude and 26°45′28″ east longitude. It is mostly vegetarian village and has a small population of 992. The size of land holdings are not big; basis of livelihood of the rural community is agriculture but, on the whole, the rural community is large enough which cannot be fed on the existing land. The agricultural efficiency is also low, with the result that most of the young males specially during off season go to the nearby towns for earning their livelihood while womenfolk work in the agricultural fields. Wheat, rice (transplanted and broadcast), peas, barley, pulses (arhar, masur), some coarse grains, melons, potatoes are the main cash crops.

The detailed survey in the different economic groups of people of the village is conducted with a view to assess the nutritional status of the rural population. This survey is spread over three seasons corresponding to summer, winter and third the rainy season.

The dietary intake information so gathered is processed and a food intake sheet per head per day is prepared (Table 5.3). Further, this type of survey has revealed the extent to which food is under-nutritive or mal-nutritive. It is found that the population is suffering from mal and to a larger extent from under-nourishment.

It is revealed from Table 5.3 the extent of caloric intake per head per day from all sources during the year 2001. It is observed that like other villages here too residents of category A take 2353 calories per head per day while the intake for categories B and C 2267 and 1777 respectively. There are, however, a few families in every village which depend on pulses only. It is observed that the main sources of calories are rice, wheat, pulses few roots and green vegetables; egg, butter, milk contributes a little, generally in categories B and C. Table further

Table 5.3 : Dhanipur : Supply of Different Nutrients per head per day in the Categories A, B, C, and percentage of Departure from Standard Requirement

Elements of Food	*Standard Requirement*	*Actual Intake* A	*Actual Intake* B	*Actual Intake* C	*PDSR* A	*PDSR* B	*PDSR* C
Protein g	68	62.4	68.7	49.8	-8.3	+1.0	-26.8
Fat g	50	52.8	47.2	33.6	+5.6	-5.6	-32.9
Carbohydrate g	440	400.6	392.0	318.0	-8.9	-10.8	-27.8
Calcium mg	700	487.5	383.2	259.9	-30.3	-45.2	-62.8
Iron mg	22.5	47.11	45.8	36.8	+109.3	+103.6	+63.4
Vitamin-A I.U.	3500	1856.0	1654.3	1569.2	-46.9	-52.7	-55.2
Thiamine mg	1.12	2.30	2.26	1.65	+105.3	101.8	+47.3
Riboflavin mg	1.46	1.56	1.35	1.1	+6.9	-7.5	-26.7
Niacin mg	19	20.1	35.0	16.1	+5.8	+84.3	-15.3
Vitamin-C mg	43	19.7	26.0	29.8	-54.2	-39.4	-30.7
Calories	2400	2353	2267	1777	-1.9	-5.5	-26.0

reveals that the total amount of various food elements consumed by an individual per head per day is unsatisfactory except in the case of iron and thiamine (+109.3 +103.6, +63.4 and +105.3, + 101.8, +47.3) respectively. For a healthy growth, it is essential to have a balanced diet which should contain all the essential nutrients in their appropriate quantity, e.g. protein, fat, carbohydrates, vitamins and minerals.

Protein is essential for normal body functioning and repair. It can be used for energy at the time of low caloric intake. It is, therefore, essential that the required quantity of protein should be taken each day by every individual. It has been observed that except category B people (+1 per cent), the remaining two categories have below average (A) –8.3 and (C) –26.8 per cent. Several important functions of metabolism depend upon fat as it helps in absorption of fat soluble vitamins as well as iron .The present survey reveals that on an average, the villagers do not get the recommended quantity of 50 gm except for people belonging to category (A) + 5.6 per cent; B and C categories are living on –5.6 and C –32.9 per cent respectively. Whereas the supply of carbohydrates are short in all categories to the level of (A) –8.9, (B) –10.8 and (C) –27.8. similar situation in regard to calcium; it is also deficient to the level of –30.3, –45.2 and –62.8 per cent respectively. Next element that counts much is vitamin-D which is received in natural course from the sun rays. As it is known, that calcium is fundamental in teeth formation, while vitamin-D increase the rate of absorption, and helps in bone calcification. Rickets is severe manifestation of deprivation of all these elements, in which bones become soft and pliable: short supply of protein and calories cause, kwashiorkor/marasmus. With the result that these shortages, 15.7 per cent cases of rickets and 7.1 per cent cases of kwashiorkor/marasmus were reported from the village Dhanipur (Fig. 5.1).

Vitamins are also equally important for the body, e.g. vitamin-A is essential for the formation and maintenance of healthy skin and membranes and is a component that enables vision in dim light, but it is very unfortunate that the population of the village lacks such important component to the level of –46.9, –52.7 and –55.2 per cent respectively and creates vision and related problems (17.8 per cent). Thiamine, riboflavin and niacin are involved in energy metabolism, thiamine acts as co-enzymes in the metabolism of carbohydrates, riboflavin is essential in oxidative systems, niacin in respiratory systems of energy metabolism.[16] Vitamin C is used to provide intercellular strength necessary for the connection of tissues but supply

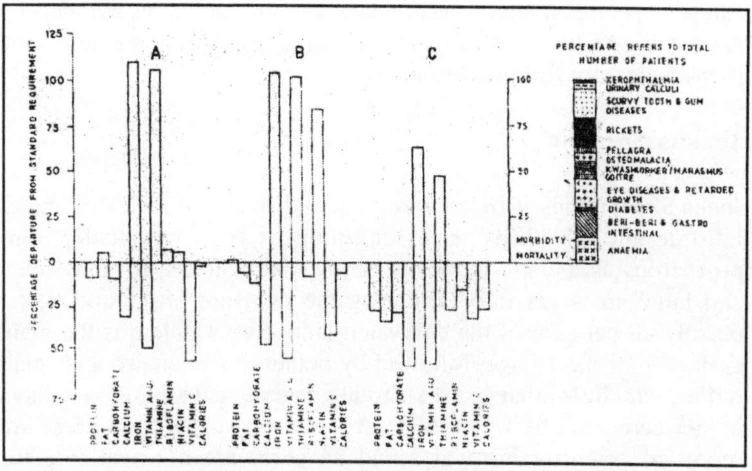

Fig. 5.1 : Nutritional Deficiency Diseases : Dhanipur

of all these vitamins with single exception of thiamine is short either in all categories or in one or two categories. This situation is due to little intake of green leavy negetables, milk or milk products, fruits on regular or routine basis. Riboflavin is short in B and D (–7.5 and –26.7 per cent) respectively while niacin is short only in (C) category –15.3 per cent. Further, vitamin-C is short in the entire village community (A) –54.2 per cent (B) –39.4 per cent and (C) –30.7 per cent. This is unique that its intake is relatively low in the higher category. The obvious reason seems to be that lower class is busy in producing vegetables and some other indigenous items of food like *mahua, jamun* and *berre*.

Survey results also reveals various types of deficiency diseases (12.3 per cent) prevalent in the village. Beri-beri/gastrointestinal disturbances, scurvy along with tooth and gum swelling problems and anaemia (14.9, 15.9 and 13.8 per cent) followed by eye diseases retarded growth. Kwashiorkor/marasmus and rickets (17.8, 7.1 and 15.7 per cent) whereas others acçount for comparatively low number of patients—osteomalacia 4,6 per cent, pellagra 3.1 per cent, urinary calculi 3.1 per cent and diabetes (Fig. 5.1). Goitre and xerophthalamia, 1.5, 2.5 and 1.5 per cent respectively. The mortality as a result of these deficiency diseases is lowest in (A) category and highest in lower economic group. The probable reason for this seems to be the availability of good food and its adequate supply. Most of the (A) category people are not forced to take certain food items but they are consuming by their choice as they can afford to some extent food items necessary for their health.

Jhakha Sheopur

Jhaka Sheopur lies at 18 km west of Musafirkhana at 26°23′10″ north latitude and 81°37′40″ east longitude. It is economically non-prosperous as the soil is mostly sandy with patches of sandy-loam and large areas get flooded during the monsoon. Rice and wheat occupy 40 per cent of the cultivated land. Sweet potato is the main cash crop of the village, followed by bejher, jowar, maize and small millets with little arhar (pulses). Total geographical area of the village is 895 acres, out of which 636 acres are un-irrigated; 68 acres are recorded as cultivable waste and 86 acres are not available for agricultural purposes. 343 males 41 females are engaged in agricultural pursuits and hence they may be called agricultural workers. The entire population of the village numbering 1856 is divided in two groups; firstly, active which comprises the agricultural workers and secondly, inactive which refers to farm owners who generally do not work in the fields.

A good portion of vitamin-C is received through fruits as they use mahua (*Bassia latifolia*) in their daily meal from the month of April; firstly, they use green mahua, and later on it is dry with mango. They also occasionally take cereals with mahua. In the off-season potato and sweet potato constitute their basic diet. In the morning they generally use the surplus left over in the early evening. Most of the calories are derived from cereals, pulses and vegetables. Seasonal fruits, meat and milk, all together contribute a little amount of calories. The daily intake of calories varies from 2669, 2046.9 to 1931.1. More than 50 per cent of the population is non-vegetarian. This village has a mixed population, Ghosies, (milkman) are in majority followed by Mallah (ferry people), Dhobi (washerman), Harijans (scheduled caste Hindus), Ahir (Hindu milkman) and Brahmns/Pandits (high caste Hindus). The consumption of milk and fish is more common in this village. Nevertheless most of the people cannot afford to buy milk, eggs, meat, fish for their daily diets. These items are either familiar with those who trade in these commodities or those who can afford to purchase them.

There is a considerable variation in the nutritional position of the villagers. Their dietary habits are also different. With the result they suffer from mal-nourishment due to continuous intake of unbalanced diet. Such diets cause several deficiency diseases among them. The relationship of faulty diet to the disease is an old story. James Lind's famous 'treatise on scurvy' was published in 1753. What were new at the 1963 Nutritional Congress, was the dietary factors in the causation of 'Cardio-vascular diseases'[17] in man. However the total number of patients in this village was 19.9 per cent out of which 73.4 per cent were suffering from deficiency diseases, viz. anaemia 13.2, beri-beri and gastro-intestinal disturbances 16.4, diabetes 4.0, eye diseases 15.6 per cent. Whereas kwashiorkor/marasmus, osteomalacia, pellagra, rickets, scurvy, tooth and gum diseases along with urinary calculi account for 6.9, 6.5, 7.2, 10.4, 18.4 and 2.7 per cent and has proved a close relationship between deficient supply of nutrients and the existing deficiency diseases in the village (Fig. 5.2)

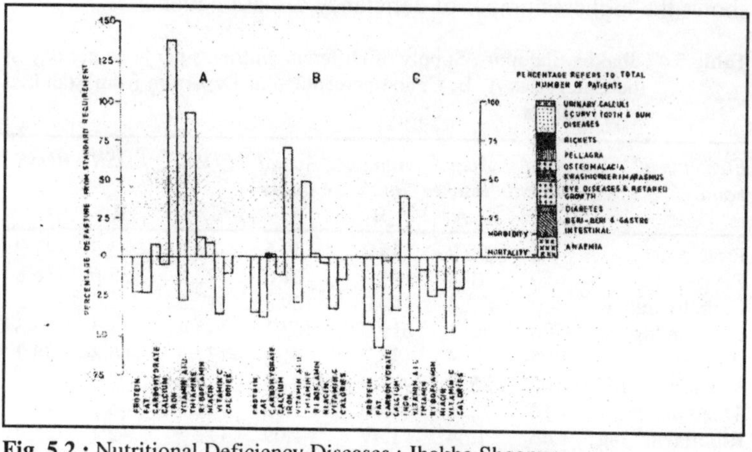

Fig. 5.2 : Nutritional Deficiency Diseases : Jhakha Sheopur

Besides the deficiency of fat, protein, calcium, the supply of calories are also deficient in categories of B and C. If the conditions are measured on the average caloric requirement of 2000 per head per day as supported by Shafi, for Eastern Uttar Pradesh,[18] even then the supply of calories in category C is short.

Supply of thiamine, iron and carbohydrate is fair but in the absence of other nutrients, they cannot ensure a good health. Morbidity and mortality rates recorded in the village during the survey is found to be 14.6 and 1.7 respectively. Table 5.4 shows the supply of fat, protein, calcium, vitamin-A and C has gone down to the tune of –22.6, –22.2, –5.4, –27.8 and –36.0 per cent in the case of category A people, whereas it is short to the tune of –37.6, 33.5, –11.5, –29.3, –32.1 per cent and –56.8, –41.9, –33.3, –46.2 and –47.9 per cent in the case of categories B and C respectively. In the village under study, people belonging to low income group (category C) suffered more than other village population. From the given Table 5.4, it is clear that there is little difference in the supply of essential nutrients among the categories A and B, although category A registered six plus and B registered four. But in category C only one plus (iron+38.7) is recorded. The supply of other nutrients are inadequate, rather far below the standard requirement.

Poor availability of food and faulty diet particularly in category C has resulted in 70 per cent of the deficiency patients in this category. The labour class becomes easy victim to these problems. This village shows the highest number of deficiency disease patients.

Table 5.4 : Jhakha-Sheopur : Supply of Different Nutrients per head per day in the Categories A, B, C, and percentage of Departure from Standard Requirement.

Elements of Food	*Standard Requirement*	*Actual Intake* A	*Actual Intake* B	*Actual Intake* C	*PDSR* A	*PDSR* B	*PDSR* C
Protein g	68	52.9	45.2	39.5	-22.2	-33.5	-41.9
Fat g	50	38.7	31.2	21.6	-22.6	-37.6	-56.8
Carbohydrate g	440	472.4	446.0	429.8	+7.5	+1.4	-2.3
Calcium mg	700	662.1	619.0	467.1	-5.4	-11.5	-33.3
Iron mg	22.5	53.4	38.1	31.2	+137.3	+69.4	+38.7
Vitamin-A I.U.	3500	2527	2474.9	1884.9	-27.8	-29.3	-46.2
Thiamine mg	1.12	2.16	1.66	1.03	+92.8	+48.2	-8.0
Riboflavin mg	1.46	1.64	1.49	1.09	+12.3	+2.1	-25.4
Niacin mg	19	20.6	18.2	14.8	+8.7	-4.2	-22.1
Vitamin-C mg	43	27.5	29.2	22.4	-36.0	-32.1	-47.9
Calories	2400	2669	2046.9	1931.1	+11.2	-14.7	-19.5

Kichaucha

The village Ashrafpur Kichaucha lies at a distance of 19 km from its tahsil Tanda in district Faizabad on Tanda-Jalalpur road and is located in 82° 45′ 45″ north latitude and 26°25′14″ east longitude. It is the famous site of Great Muslim 'Sufi' Saint Ashraf Jahangir Samnani. It is inhabited by his muslim descendents and as well as by Hindus, comprising mostly of Kewats and Harijans (Scheduled Castes).

The village is very well connected by road. It still has many ponds and streams linking each other which often overflow during the rainy season, particularly western flank of the villages is ill-drained and gives often one crop while the eastern flank is better and produces good rice crops, sugarcane and also wheat production is normal. Peas, gram, maize cover very little area but pulses and small millets are grown on regular basis. Besides sugarcane, potato is another cash crop which is produced on limited scale whereas in the neighboring areas potato and sugarcane are highly remunerative. The village has 15 tube-wells and 11 tractors but the owners are generally not holding much land that can justify the investment. Since the farmers extend such facilities to others on hire basis on these items. It has been seen that tractors are used in this village on a small scale for agricultural and related works, while in off-season, they are used for non-agricultural pursuits, e.g. transportation of bricks, earth for filling depression, carrying the passengers and using it at the time of marriage.

Approximately 40 per cent of the total population 9148 is Muslim and the rest consists of non-Muslims. About 70 per cent of the non-Muslim population is non-vegetarian. Muslims are generally land owners and their holdings vary from one acre to 6 acres. They do not entirely depend on agriculture alone but do some other work to increase the income, e.g. (A) category includes some muslims who are considered as Peers (religious heads); they use to travel widely among their followers and get lot of money as gifts and hence they can meet their requirements even without any income from lands and some are known as khadims and mujabirs associated with tomb of Makhdoum Syed Ashraf Jahangir. But in other communities, about 70 per cent are agricultural workers (Harijans and Kewats). They work during the sowing and harvesting seasons and do some extra work in the off-season e.g. they work as rickshaw pullers, and some of them as labourers in construction work.

There is a Government Ayurvedic dispensary, a biweekly market, (Thursday and Sunday). On the market day meat, fish and fresh vegetables are available.

As usual, houses of the flower starta are of mud with thatched roof or part is covered with khaprail (mud tiles); whereas the middle class has more than one room for living, made of mud and bricks covered with khaprail roofs. The (A) category people possess large-sized rooms made of bricks and cement, most of them have electric connections too.

Majority of the population is non-vegetarian, but like other villages, availability of necessary nutrients are not satisfactory. In the first instance, where they can afford they are not aware of the concept of balanced diet; rather they go by choices bases on tradition or taste. Secondly, those who cannot afford to have such diets, are not aware of its importance, otherwise they might have tried within their limited means atleast to improve the daily intake. There are some families who are not in a position to feed their members even two times a day during difficult period of the season. The category (C) which needs much calories is getting the lowest calories (1854). As stated earlier, the caloric intake varies according to the nature of work performed. Considering 2400 calories per head per day as the standard for this area, it is observed that the daily intake is short by 84, 256 and 546 in the three categories respectively.

Table 5.5 shows the nutritional level of the rural communities in the three categories, i.e. A, B and C. About 7 per cent of the population still suffers from under-nutrition and the morbidity rate during the survey was assessed at 11.8 per cent with 1.4 per cent as mortality rate. Among the most prevalent deficiency diseases are beri-beri, sciatica, gastro-intestinal disturbances, colitis (16.4 per cent), followed by Scurvy, tooth and gum diseases (18.6 per cent) and pellagra, rickets

Table 5.5 : Kichaucha : Supply of Different Nutrients per head per day in the Categories A, B, C, and percentage of Departure from Standard Requirement

Elements of Food	*Standard Requirement*	*Actual Intake* A	*Actual Intake* B	*Actual Intake* C	*PDSR* A	*PDSR* B	*PDSR* C
Protein g	68	85.4	60.7	62.2	+25.5	-10.7	-8.5
Fat g	50	96.7	22.3	27.3	+93.4	-55.4	-45.3
Carbohydrate g	440	446.2	414.3	331.7	+1.4	-5.8	-24.6
Calcium mg	700	721.5	722.4	1062.4	+3.1	+3.2	-51.8
Iron mg	22.5	29.3	29.8	39.8	+30.2	+32.4	+76.8
Vitamin-A I.U.	3500	2878.9	2104.5	3597.2	-17.7	-39.9	+2.8
Thiamine mg	1.12	1.34	1.64	2.23	+19.6	+46.4	+99.1
Riboflavin mg	1.46	1.18	1.25	1.45	-19.2	-14.4	-0.68
Niacin mg	19	23.4	21.8	18.42	+23.1	+14.7	-3.1
Vitamin-C mg	43	36.6	18.6	41.9	-14.9	-56.7	-2.5
Calories	2400	2316	2144.0	1854	-3.5	-10.6	-22.8

(12.2, 6.8 per cent) respectively. Kwashiorkor, marasmus or fatty heirs also accounts for 6.7 per cent in the village. Anaemia, eye diseases, retarded growth, keratomalacia, urinary calculi, diabetes, osteomalacia and goitre accounts for 9.9, 10.9, 2.0, 7.1, 3.3, 4.2 and 1.9 per cent respectively (Fig. 5.3).

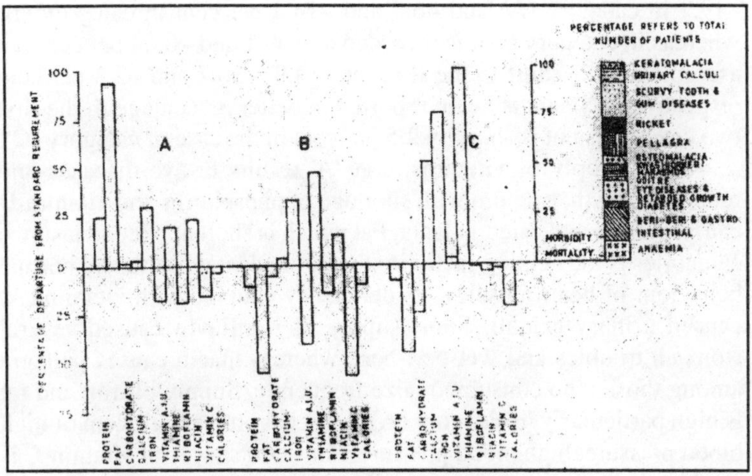

Fig. 5.3 : Nutritional Deficiency Diseases : Kichaucha

The supply of different nutrients are not uniformly distributed among the different categories of inhabitants; they vary from category to category, viz. the supply of first three elements protein, fat and carbohydrate is short in the last two categories to the tune of (–10.7, –8.5, –55.4, –45.3 and –5.8, –24.6 per cent) respectively. Whereas its supply is in surplus i.e. +25.5, +93.4 and +1.4 per cent in the category A people. The supply of iron and calcium is fairly good in all the categories (+30.2, + 32.4, +76.8 and +3.1, +3.2, +51.8 per cent respectively). However, vitamin–A is available satisfactorily in (C) category, i.e. 2.8 per cent but its shortage is reported in the other two categories (A) –17.7 per cent and in (B) –39.9 per cent. The obvious reason for good supply of calcium and vitamin-A in (C) category is due to frequent use of fish and vegetables by the kewats (scheduled caste) and Muslims of the area and its low supply relatively in (A) category is caused by the absence of leafly vegetables and fish, by and large they opt for meat in place of these two items.

It is clear from Table 5.5 that the nutritional position is not very sound. It deteriorates from A to B and C. Consequently the villagers belonging to groups (B) and (C) are more prone to deficiency diseases in comparison to category (A) people. Occurrence of these diseases is closely associated with the existing supply level of nutrients.

The actual supply of vitamins thiamine and riboflavin is –19.6, –19.2 in category (A) and 46.4 and –14.4 per cent in category (B) whereas in category C, it is recorded as +99.1 and –0.68 per cent but ascorbic acid is short to the level of –14.9, –56.7 and –2.5 per cent respectively. Niacin is again reported in better percentage in the first two categories but is short by 2.5 per cent in the case of category (C).

Short supply of vitamins, e.g. 'A' results in eye diseases and retarded growth; calcium with shortage of phosphorus and vitamin-D causes rickets and osteomalacia. Fat which is short applied in last two categories is the helping factor in disturbing dental health and normal behaviour of heart muscles. Its deficiency coupled with vitamin (A) caused urinary calculi. Short supply of riboflavin caused several stomach troubles and wet beri-beri, whereas niacin causes pellagra among those who consume maize frequently. Supply of iron and fat is high particularly in category (A) that it has created problem of high blood pressure; high blood pressure with short supply of vitamin-C is more dangerous as it may hamper blood clotting and body resistance. It may cause scurvy, tooth and gum diseases.

Protein supply is short in 'B' and 'C' categories with the result that kwashiorkor/marasmus is common. Protein deficiency with short calories cause marasmus. So merely getting some nutrient in surplus does not mean that certain disease would not occur, their occurrence very much depends on other factors too.

Khizrabad

Khizrabad is a small village with total population of 308, 140 males and 168 females; total area of the village is 157 acres. The village lies in 26°11′ 00″ north latitude and 82°22′00″ east longitude at a distance of about 4 km to the north-west of Kadipur tahsil headquarter in Sultanpur district.

The village of Khizrabad is situated along the high bank of river Gomati, a perennial stream meandering towards the west and a strip of 11 acres of land goes along with it. Which is not available for cultivation due to heavy erosion. The village is also not well-connected;

an unmetalled road between Dostpur and Kadipur passes at a distance of 2 km from the village.

Predominant soil of the village is sandy-loam but patches of sandy soil can also be seen. Irrigation facilities are very poor with the result that 94 out of 157 acres of land are almost left unirrigated. The existing means of irrigations are also very old. Wheat and gram are the staple rabi crops; in the kharif, 92 per cent of the land is covered by broad cast rice; next is the big millets mixed with pulses (arhar). Only one acre of land is registered as cultivable waste in 2001.

The village is inhabited by various communities and naturally dietary habits are also different. There are only some (A) class families and the rest belong to (B) and (C) categories people.

Majority of the village population is mal-nourished supply of necessary nutrients in their diet is inadequate in all the categories, but varies in the quantity such as the supply of calories among the people of all the three categories are short by –3.5 per cent in (A), –10.6 and –22.8 per cent in B and C categories per head per day (Table 5.6). Main sources of supply are cereals and about 85 per cent of the population is unable to reach the target of the standard intake of 2400 per person per day. The supply of protein, fat alongwith riboflavin, niacin and vitamin-C is not upto the mark with the result that 12.7 per cent of the villagers are liable to various deficiency diseases.

Table 5.6 : Khizrabad : Supply of Different Nutrients per head per day in the Categories A, B, C, and percentage of Departure from Standard Requirement

Elements of Food	*Standard Requirement*	*Actual Intake* A	*Actual Intake* B	*Actual Intake* C	*PDSR* A	*PDSR* B	*PDSR* C
Protein g	68	65.4	60.7	62.2	-3.8	-10.7	-8.5
Fat g	50	36.7	22.3	27.3	-26.5	-55.4	-45.3
Carbohydrate g	440	446.2	414.3	331.7	+1.4	-5.8	-24.6
Calcium mg	700	571.6	722.0	1062.4	-18.3	+3.2	+51.8
Iron mg	22.5	29.3	39.8	49.2	+30.0	+76.8	+118.8
Vitamin-A I.U.	3500	1878.9	2104.5	3597.2	-46.3	-39.9	+2.8
Thiamine mg	1.12	1.34	1.64	2.23	+9.8	+34.4	+82.8
Riboflavin mg	1.46	1.18	1.25	1.45	-19.2	-14.4	-0.68
Niacin mg	19	23.4	21.8	18.4	+23.0	+14.9	-3.1
Vitamin-C mg	43	26.6	18.6	41.9	-38.1	-56.8	-2.5
Calories	2400	2316	2144.6	1853.2	-3.5	-10.6	-22.8

The most common among them are beri-beri and gastro-intestinal, colitis etc. Deficiency diseases above account for 12.7 per cent of the total patients with 1.9 per cent morality (Fig. 5.4). As most of the deficiency diseases are not killer, even then create problems by making the people inactive and spoiling normal functioning of the body mechanism and if prolonged, may end up with death or render inactive by paralising any part of the body.

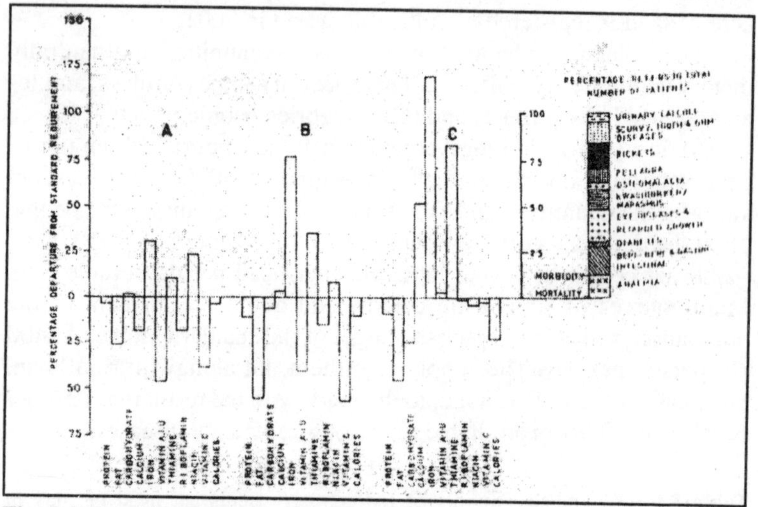

Fig. 5.4 : Nutritional Deficiency Diseases : Khizrabad

It is clear from the Table 5.6 that the nutritional status of the villagers is far from satisfactory and the supply of various food elements is not uniform, viz. the supply of iron, thiamine, to some extent protein, niacin, calcium and riboflavin is fairly well in all the three categories in comparison to the supply of fat and vitamin-C which are deficient to the tune of –26.5, –38.1 respectively in the families of (A) category and –55.4, –56.8 in case of (B) category whereas in (C), these figures are –45.3, –2.5 per cent respectively per head per day. While the shortage of carbohydrates is recorded only in B and C categories (–5.8 and –24.60 per cent), the supply of vitamin-A is short in category (A) and (B) to the tune of –46.3 and –39.3 respectively. Generalised use of fish and leafy vegetables and seasonal fruits which are not normally used in category A, are the main source of vitamin-C in category (B) and (C).

There is no custom of taking refined table salt or bathing with seasalt, therefore, the distribution of iodine and vitamin-D is almost even in all three categories as for both they depend on nature. Out of the total population of the village, 12.7 per cent are sick, majority belongs to C and B categories. Beri-beri, gastro-intestinal problems, retarded/stunted growth and eye diseases, scurvy/tooth and gum diseases. Kwashiorkor/marasmus and pellagra together account about 64.7 per cent of the total deficiency patients. Due to the deficient supply of riboflavin, thiamine among category (C) people. 15.6 per cent of the patients registered complaints of gastro-intestinal trouble, colitis in the age groups of old people and young children have the symptoms of beri-beri. Sciatica is also noticed in developed and semi-developed form. While scurvy, tooth and gum problems and kwashiorkor/marasmus account for 11.6 per cent and 11.5 per cent respectively, due to acute shortage of vitamin-C in A and B categories. In adequate supply of protein, fat along with low caloric intake causes kwashiorkor/marasmus and also results in poor heir conditions. Pellagra is the diseases which is associated with the niacin deficiency. Though niacin is not much short, even then 8.1 per cent kids have the developed symptoms of pellagra. Deficiency of vitamin-A and D claims for 17.9 and 12.8 per cent of patients suffering from different eye diseases, retarded growth and rickets. Short supply of fat creates hindrance in absorbing fat soluble vitamins.

The supply of iron and thiamine is surplus in all the categories. Due to non-absorption in the body or unusual discharge of blood from the body, deficiency may develop, several cases of anaemia also reported (12.8 per cent). Besides these diseases, other diseases are also noticed among the rural community, i.e. diabetes, urinary calculi and osteomalacia is found at the rate of 2.5, and 3.2 per cent respectively (Fig. 5.5). Although the village is not agriculturally developed, yet the supply of essential food elements is better due to additional seasonal availability of wild vegetables, fruits and fish especially to the downtrodden society. No case of goitre, xerophthalmia, keratomalacia is reported from this village.

Ariya Bazar

Village Ariya of tahsil Akberpur, district Ambedkar Nagar, is situated at 26^{0} 29′23″ north latitide and 82^{0} 35′21″ east longitude. It is located at a distance of 5.5 km from Akbarpur on either side of Akbarpur-Tanda road and lies on Khadar land. Sarda canal passing through this village is a good source of irrigation beside three ponds, tube-wells and wells.

The village is very well connected with other neighboring villages of the area. A metalled road connects the village to the railway station lying at a distance of 1 km at Surapur. The village has a government dispensary and a market.

About 79 per cent of the total land is under cultivation, out of which 90 per cent is devoted to grain crops, wheat occupies the largest percentage. It is sown as a single crop as well as in combination with barley and mustard. Wheat is often sown in the fields left fallow during the Kharif season. Peas, gram, mustard are seldom sown as a sole crop. Rice (broadcast and transplanted) occupies major portion followed by small millets and sugarcane in the kharif season. On the whole about 70 per cent of the land is devoted to double cropping.

Cereals constitutes the major portion of food of the people like other villages and provide more than 70 per cent of their caloric intake. Total population of the village (1802 persons) is comprised of baniyas (traders), Muslims and scheduled castes. Meat and fish is consumed by only Muslims in general but a section of non-Muslims also generally go for meat in weekly market. However, mutton, eggs, fish, milk products are not within the reach of every person. Vegetable (root and leafy) are the main source of vitamins and calcium. Oils and fats are not available at a satisfactory level.

Table 5.7 reveals the extent of caloric intake per head per day from all sources available during 2001. It is observed that categories A and B have higher caloric intake with 2696.3 and 2362 than category C, which has 1971.7 per head per day. The mortality rate recorded in the village is 10.5 and 1.4 per cent respectively. In category A families have a surplus of all essential nutrients except vitamin A and C which is short to the level of –20.8 and –34.7 as is also the case of other two categories where the shortage is –53.5, –44.3, –6.9, and –26.2 per cent. It is also obvious that total amount of various food elements consumed by categories B and C are unsatisfactory except in the case of calcium, iron, riboflavin and niacin (+16.1, +175.6, +46.4, +10.9 and +8.9 respectively) in category B. Iron and thiamine are the only surplus nutrients in the diets of category C people (+93.3 +59.8). Majority of population belongs to category C which are generally living under conditions of mal and under-nutrition. Category A people as represent small section of population and often suffer from mal-nutrition or lacking a balanced diet.

Table 5.7 : Ariya Bazar : Supply of Different Nutrients per head per day in the Categories A, B, C, and percentage of Departure from Standard Requirement

Elements of Food	*Standard Requirement*	*Actual Intake* A	*Actual Intake* B	*Actual Intake* C	*PDSR* A	*PDSR* B	*PDSR* C
Protein g	68	93.6	65.6	56.11	+37.6	-3.5	-17.5
Fat g	50	66.6	37.2	56.1	+33.2	-25.6	-57.6
Carbohydrate g	440	533.2	389.2	21.2	+21.2	-11.5	-18.0
Calcium mg	700	881.7	812.6	360.7	+25.9	+16.1	- 43.7
Iron mg	22.5	53.8	62.0	43.5	+139.1	+175.6	+93.3
Vitamin-A I.U.	3500	2772.0	1628.6	43.5	-20.8	-53.5	-44.3
Thiamine mg	1.12	1.63	1.64	1951.1	+45.5	+46.4	+59.8
Riboflavin mg	1.46	1.73	1.62	1.79	+18.5	+10.9	-9.6
Niacin mg	19	21.3	20.7	1.32	+12.7	+8.9	-4.3
Vitamin-C mg	43	28.1	40.04	18.2	-34.7	-6.9	-26.2
Calories	2400	2696.3	2362.0	1971.7	+12.2	-1.6	-17.8

Protein is essential for a normal body function and its supply although short in least two categories B and C, is not very low–3.5 in B and –17.5 per cent in C. The position of fat which is a supporting element of food is again bad with –25.6 and –57.6 per cent in categories B and C respectively Calcium supply is exceptionally good in A and B atleast, and short in category C by –43.7 per cent. Distribution of carbo hydrates is also not even as category A has positive supply +21.2 per cent, whereas last two categories B and C has negative reading –11.5 and 18.0 per cent respectively. Beside these nutrients position of vitamin-C is also bad but not as low as, it is found generally in other villages.

The status of iodine in water is deficient causing mal-functioning of thyroid glands and also affects vision and development of mind and body. In this village 1.5 per cent of the total deficiency patients are attributed to goitre of the total deficiency patients are attributed to goitre.

The percentage of occurrence of various diseases is high where the intake of iodine is below the recommend level. Even in categories where the caloric intake or intake of some of the other nutrients are normal or above, the spread of nutritional deficiency diseases cannot altogether be ruled out. The major diseases found among the villagers are scurvy/tooth and gum disease (16.1 per cent), beri-beri gastro-intestinal disturbances colitis, etc. (14.6 per cent). Although the supply of iron is in surplus but the cases of anaemia (11.5 per cent) are also evident, may be because of non-absorption or loss of blood due to reasons explained earlier. Eye diseases stunted, retarded growth, xerophthalmia and kerotomalacia (12.8, 3.0 and 2.5 per cent), rickets kwashiorkor/marasmus, pellagra and urinary calculi (9.2, 7.6, 6.8 and 6.1 per cent), are other diseases noticed in this village. A low percentage of diabetes (4.8 per cent), and osteomalacia (3.5 per cent) is also noted in the village (Fig. 5.5). Further it has been seen that the population belonging to the middle more from these diseases than those of upper starta (category A). in the present economic setup, it is rather impossible for most of the rural population to make a balanced diet.

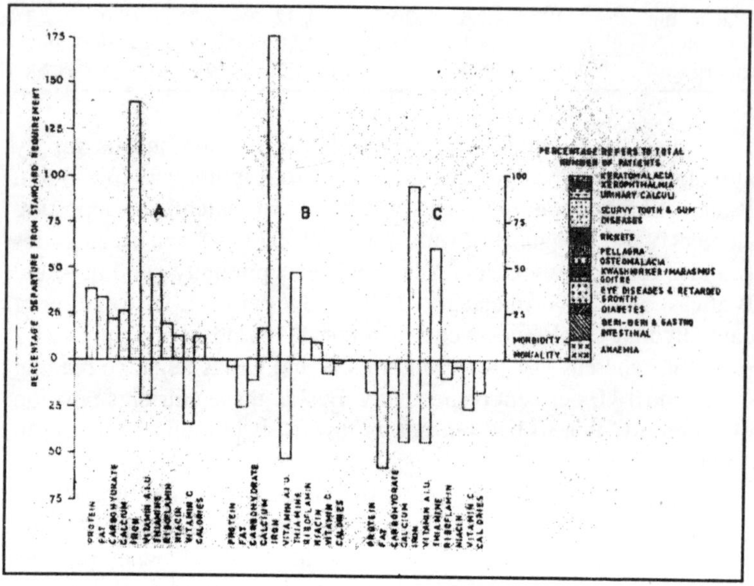

Fig. 5.5 : Nutritional Deficiency Diseases : Ariya Bazar

Dasrathpur

Village Dasrathpur lying in a well drained fertile loamy soil on Jalalpur road, 4 km away from Bikapur and to the west of Ramdaspur Majhouli is located at 26°37′15″ north latitude and 82°08′59″ east longitude. Its total area is 476 acres and it carries a population of 1449, Brahmins and Harijans (scheduled caste), represent 70 per cent of the total population, while the rest are Yadav and others.

Main agricultural crops of kharif season are rice, jowar, arhar, fodder (*chari*) and sugarcane and in rabi, wheat occupies first place followed by peas, gram, moong, and potato. Wheat and rice together occupy 346 acres of land of which 92 acres were unirrigated. The total wasteland extends over 7 acres, and the land not available for cultivation accounted for 55 acres. Villagers are in little touch with the modern agricultural development, and do not believe in statement of agricultural experts, rather they go by their own experience with the result, that the loss of fertilizer is common and also its concentration due to high doses may damage plant cells. Besides, the excessive water and fertilizer make the condition suitable for pests and diseases in the absence of required checks. Finally, the chemicals available to combat these diseases are often given after their expiry date.

The use of high yielding varieties of seeds like sonalika, arjun, janak, kalyan, sona and rice of jai, saket 4, ratna gives better results only with the help of natural and irrigation water, but transplanting must be over by 15th July, otherwise it is recommended to increase the amount of fertilizer and seedlinks.

The area which is not under cultivation (*usar* lands) can be reclaimed through applying gypsum, sulphur or lime with plenty of water to neutralize the salt, even if filled with water and waste mango leaves and left to decay, it will be cured but since the water table is high, it may destroy again if left uncultivated.

On the whole this village is well supplied with food needed. The caloric consumption per head per day varies from 2452 to 2061 most of which are derived from the cereals, especially wheat and rice. Use of vegetable and milk is more frequent in category A than in the categories B and C. Oils and fats are not available to satisfactory degree and same is the case with protein except in category A (+36.2 per cent). The supply of calcium is low (–33.7, –36.2 and –58.6 per cent) in categories A, B and C and the cases of its deficiency are high with a percentage of 11.7 and 4.9. Calcium deficiency leads to rickets which are associated with children whereas osteomalacia is found among adults. Unlike protein carbohydrates are also in short supply in the categories B and C (–5.0 and –8.9 per cent) whereas it is in surplus in category A (+3.9 per cent) as shown in Table 5.8.

Although there is a surplus of thiamine, riboflavin is short in categories B and C. The cases of beri-beri, angular stomatitis and

Table 5.8 : Dasrathpur : Supply of Different Nutrients per head per day in the Categories A, B, C, and percentage of Departure from Standard Requirement

Elements of Food	*Standard Requirement*	*Actual Intake* A	*Actual Intake* B	*Actual Intake* C	*PDSR* A	*PDSR* B	*PDSR* C
Protein g	68	92.6	59.7	49.79	+36.2	-12.2	-26.8
Fat g	50	46.6	41.4	37.5	-6.8	-17.2	-25.0
Carbohydrate g	440	457.4	417.9	400.56	+3.9	-5.02	-8.9
Calcium mg	700	464.2	446.8	209.8	-33.7	-36.2	- 58.6
Iron mg	22.5	52.1	54.7	46.9	+131.5	+143.1	+108.4
Vitamin-A I.U.	3500	4421.6	2361.2	1569.2	+26.33	-32.5	-55.2
Thiamine mg	1.12	2.35	1.82	1.65	+109.8	+62.5	+47.3
Riboflavin mg	1.46	1.95	1.14	1.40	+33.56	+-21.9	-4.1
Niacin mg	19	24.23	19.69	16.09	+27.6	+3.6	-15.3
Vitamin-C mg	43	51.3	36.8	21.04	+19.3	-14.4	-51.1
Calories	2400	2432	2452	2061	+1.33	+2.2	-14.1

chronic diarrhoea, constipation are found in this village at the prevalence rate of 16.1 per cent. This may be because of uneven distribution or extra heating or indigestion, which may have reduced its percentage in the body. Niacin is also short to the tune of –15.3 but keeping in mind the supply of this vitamin, the cases of pellagra are quite high (8.1 per cent). The short supply of protein and calories resulted in 9.9 per cent cases of kwashiorkor/marasmus.

Though iron is available in surplus like other villages anaemia is also identified (10.9 per cent). Vitamin-A and C have contributed to the eye diseases and related problems at the rate of 12.3 per cent, and xerophthalmia 2.0 per cent, while scurvy, tooth and gum diseases accounted for 14.0 per cent. These two vitamins which play an important role are both short in categories B and C. Further more vitamins-A absorption depends on fat, as it is fat soluble vitamins. Other disease recorded in this village is urinary calculi with 5.6 per cent. No iodine deficiency is reported in the year 2001.

Fig. 5.6 shows that the village, during the year of survey has 9.6 per cent morbidity and 1.04 per cent mortality rate which though not the lowest, is low among the villages under study.

Gaura-Baremau

Gaura-Baremau of block Baldiral, tahsil Musafirkhana, district

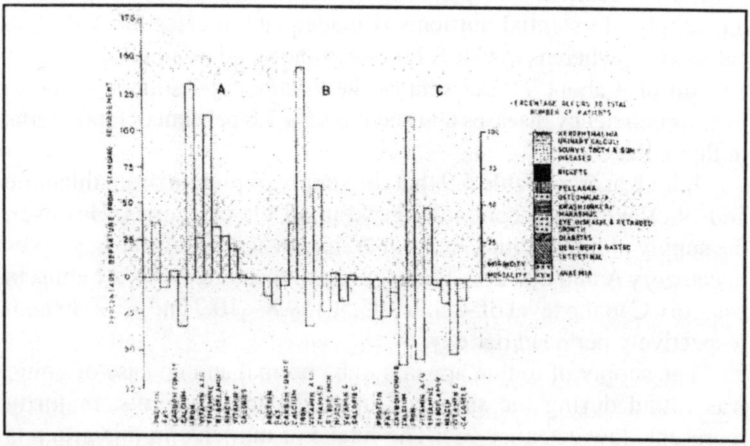

Fig. 5.6 : Nutritional Deficiency Diseases : Dasrathpur

Sultanpur lies at 26°28′03″ north latitude and 81°51′21″ east longitude and occupies fertile level land of bhangar soils. The village spreads over an area of 300 acres out of which 70 per cent is level and 30 per cent undulated plain. Rice is the leading kharif crop and wheat dominates in the rabi, followed by barely, gram, peas, sugarcane, and potato. Sweet potatoes are also grown as a cash crop in the village.

The population of this village is estimated at 1546 persons of which 20 per cent are Muslims, 5.0 per cent Thakurs, 2.0 per cent Pandits, 26.0 per cent Harijans and the rest are Ahirs (milk man) and Kurmies (vagitable grower). Agricultural efficiency of this village is good, but the supply of calories and carbohydrates is not well (+3.2, –7.7, –21.8 and 0.9, –5.5, –16.9 per cent) in the village. Cereals are the main source of these food elements. The supply of protein is good in all the three categories with the only exception of a little shortage of –1.8 in category C. The intake of fat is fairly good among the people of category A (+9.2 per cent), but it has a negative reading in categories B and C at the tune of –36.6 and –58.2 per cent respectively.

The dietary habits of the village population is mixed, vegetarian and non-vegetarian. The upper strata is comprised of Muslims and Thakurs who are non-vegetarian and, therefore, meat is a familiar food item in the village.

There is a variation in the intake of nutritive diets among the members of different village communities as shown in Table 5.9, but this variation is very well marked among the rural population belonging to different economic groups. This may be explained by the fact that the supply of essential nutrients is inadequate in category A than in category B, whereas in C it is far below the standard requirement. As a result of it about 9.0 per cent of the village population is prone to various deficiency diseases and accounts for 1.6 per cent of total deaths in this village.

It is clear from Table 5.9 that the supply of protein, iron, thiamine and riboflavin is exceptionally good in all the categories. However, the supply of fat, calcium, vitamin-A, niacin and vitamin-C is surplus in category A and niacin in B category. All these elements are short in category C to the level of –58.2, –65.5, –59.8, –10.7 and 45.9 per cent respectively per head per day.

The supply of iodine appears to be normal and no case of goitre was found during the survey. Out of the total patients, majority represents low category (C). The intake of nutrients in this group is

Table 5.9 : Gaura-Baremau : Supply of Different Nutrients per head per day in the Categories A, B, C and percentage of Departure from Standard Requirement.

Elements of Food	*Standard Requirement*	*Actual Intake* A	*Actual Intake* B	*Actual Intake* C	*PDSR* A	*PDSR* B	*PDSR* C
Protein g	68	73.26	74.00	66.74	+7.7	+8.8	-1.8
Fat g	50	54.6	31.7	20.88	+9.2	-36.6	-58.2
Carbohydrate g	440	436.2	415.73	365.48	-0.9	-5.5	-16.9
Calcium mg	700	508.3	442.2	241.3	-27.38	-36.8	- 65.5
Iron mg	22.5	51.1	52.4	32.13	+127.1	+132.8	+42.8
Vitamin-A I.U.	3500	6189.1	2793.83	1416.4	+76.83	-20.2	-59.8
Thiamine mg	1.12	2.2	2.2	2.4	+80.32	+80.34	+96.7
Riboflavin mg	1.46	2.1	1.92	1.97	+43.83	+31.5	+34.9
Niacin mg	19	21.4	19.96	16.96	+12.63	+5.1	-10.7
Vitamin-C mg	43	84.3	31.56	23.26	96.04	-26.6	-45.9
Calories	2400	2477.5	2215.9	1876.7	+3.2	-7.7	-21.8

inadequate. This imbalance has ultimately led to the spread of several deficiency diseases among the rural community (Fig 5.7). Anaemia, beri-beri, rickets together with scurvy/tooth and gum diseases, accounted for more than 50 per cent of the patients. The cases of anaemia (12.2 per cent) are reported from all groups, Where as beri-beri/gastro-intestinal disturbances (13.5 per cent) are mainly contributed by category C, while the cases of rickets, scurvy/tooth

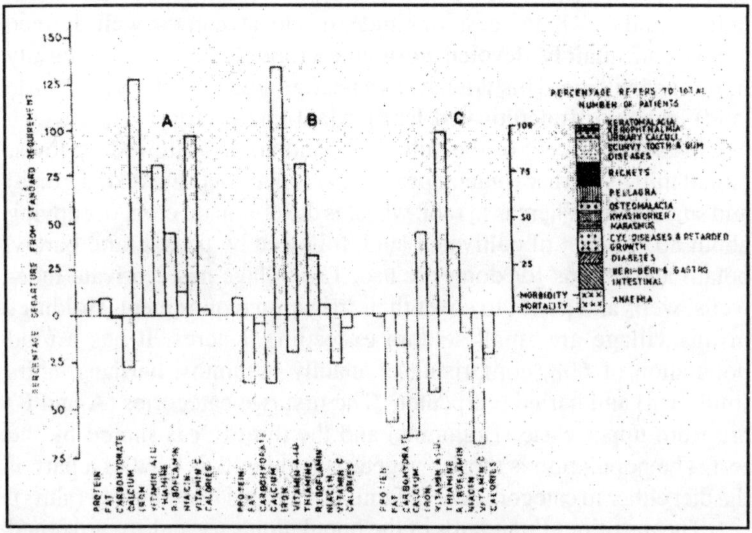

Fig. 5.7 : Nutritional Deficiency Diseases : Gaura Baremau

and gum diseases accounts for 12.5, 13.1 per cent respectively in the village. Vitamin-C has an important role in protecting people from eye diseases, and dry beri-beri and helping them in their mental development. Its deficiency may create many-fold problems for human health. It is deficient in the categories B and C to the tune of –20.2 and –59.9 per cent, resulting in 10.6, 1.5 per cent of the patients suffering from night blindness, colour blindness, retarded growth, xerophthalmia and keratomalacia. Its deficiency alongwith acute deficiency of calcium and fat caused osteomalacia and urinary calculi (4.6, 4.1 per cent).

Besides these deficiency diseases, there are pellagra, kwashiorkor/ marasmus and diabetes. Short supply of group B vitamins further leads to constipation, anorexia nervous irritability, depression, etc. A prolonged deficiency of niacin, protein and calories helps the causation of pellagra, kwashiorkor/marasmus (9.2, 10.8 per cent). Diabetes accounted for 6.4 per cent of the total deficiency patients in the village (Fig. 5.7).

Ramnathpur

The village Ramathpur lies at a distance of 1 km from Amethi in the district Sultanpur, on the Amethi-Sultanpur road and 26°10′26″ north latitude and 81°48′36″ east longitude. It is located in the well-drained loamy soil, mainly devoted to double crops. It is an agriculturally developed village. This village has a negligible area under *usar* (waste land) or banjar (uncultivated land). Main kharif crop is rice, which occupies 60 per cent of the cultivated land and is followed by jowar (small millets), arhar (pigeon pea), *chari* (big millets harvested green) and sugarcane. Whereas in rabi, wheat is the dominant crop, occupying about 80 per cent of cultivated land, followed by peas, gram, barely, potato and onions for domestic use. The village has 2 private tube-wells, wells and ponds to cover their irrigation requirement. Holdings in this village are small seldom exceeding 7 acres. It has a total population of 608, comprising of mainly brahmins, harijans, ahirs (milkman) and barhai (carpenter). The first two categories (A and B) are from upper caste (Brahmins) and the third (C) is shared by the rest. The population is mostly vegetarian and milk is used as a part of the diet either in category A or in families engaged in milk trade (ahirs).

The nutritional standards of the population vary and are governed mainly by the economic status of an individual family. Cereals and pulses normally contribute the basic diet of the inhabitants, supplemented by vegetables, milk and seasonal fruits. Pulses are main source of protein supply.

Nutritional position of the villagers has been assessed by considering the dietary habits. This is based on the supply of different essential nutrients and their percentage departure from the standard requirement. Caloric intake of the village population per head per day varies from 2520 in category A, 2289 in category B to 1988 in category C.

More than 80 per cent of the population is unable to get the required calories of 2400 per head per day. The supply of different nutrients are not uniformly distributed among the rural inhabitants. It varies from one economic category to another category, viz., the supply of protein and fat is fair, the supply of iron, vitamin-A, thiamine, riboflavin and vitamin-C is surplus, and the supply of carbohydrates, calcium and niacin is upto some extent satisfactory in category A. The supply of protein, fat, calcium and vitamin-A is deficient in categories B and C (–21.1, –30.7, –47.9, –52.8 and –12.3, –58.6, –48.6 and –68.9 per cent respectively, whereas the supply of carbohydrates in these categories are almost satisfactory. Supply of vitamin-C is exceptionally well in this village, due to frequent use of leafy vegetables and seasonal fruits available on the road sides trees or in village itself. Unlike category A thiamine iron is also sufficient in B and C (+44.3, 141.7 and +68.0, 100.4 respectively). As regards riboflavin and niacin, the first is fairly available only in category A, while it is short in the categories B and C (–12.3 and –17.8 per cent). Niacin is short in categories A and B (–1.8 and –6.0 per cent). It is clear from Table 5.10 that the nutritional position is not satisfactory and deteriorates from A to C categories. Consequently, villagers of these last two categories are more prone to the deficiency disease. This situation altogether accounted for 11.8 per cent of the deficiency diseases patients with per cent mortality rate (Fig. 5.8).

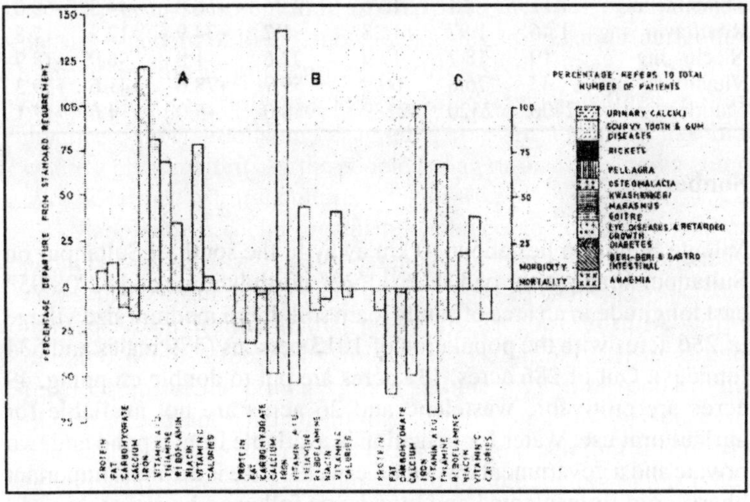

Fig. 5.8 : Nutritional Deficiency Diseases : Ramnathpur

The most common deficiency diseases in the village are beri-beri, gastrointestinal disturbances, colitis, kwashiorkor/marasmus, scurvy, tooth and gum diseases, rickets, anaemia and eye disease, which accounted for about 12.7, 12.2, 11.6, 11.3, 10.6 and 10.2 per cent respectively of the total patients in this village. Apart from these deficiency diseases pellagra, urinary-calculi, osteomalacia, diabetes and goitre are also reported and accounts for 31.4 per cent of the total patients. Due to better average supply of vitamin-A the cases of xeraphthalmia and keratomalacia are not found.

Table 5.10 : Ramnathpur : Supply of Different Nutrients per head per day in the Categories A, B, C, and percentage of Departure from Standard Requirement

Elements of Food	*Standard Requirement*	*Actual Intake* A	*Actual Intake* B	*Actual Intake* C	*PDSR* A	*PDSR* B	*PDSR* C
Protein g	68	74.3	53.6	59.6	+9.3	-21.1	-12.3
Fat g	50	56.8	34.7	20.7	+13.5	-30.7	-58.2
Carbohydrate g	440	392.3	425.0	430.3	-10.8	-3.4	-2.2
Calcium mg	700	588.8	364.1	260.1	-15.9	-47.9	- 48.6
Iron mg	22.5	49.8	54.4	45.1	+121.3	+141.7	+100.4
Vitamin-A I.U.	3500	6323.6	1651.2	1087.4	+80.7	-52.8	-68.9
Thiamine mg	1.12	2.1	1.76	2.05	+68.8	+44.3	+68.0
Riboflavin mg	1.46	1.97	1.28	1.2	+34.9	-12.3	-17.8
Niacin mg	19	18.7	17.9	22.6	-1.8	-6.0	+18.9
Vitamin-C mg	43	76.8	60.9	59.9	+78.6	+41.6	+39.3
Calories	2400	2520	2289	1988.0	+5.0	-4.6	-17.1

Sonbarsa

Village Sonbarsa lies about 10 km away to the south of Sultanpur on Sultanpur-Pratapgarh road at 26°11′22″ north latitude and 82°08′05″ east longitude in an area of sandy loam soil. It is a medium size village of 286 acres with the population of 1013 persons (479 males and 534 females). Out of 286 acres, 131 acres are put to double cropping, 49 acres are cultivable wasteland and 26 acres are not available for agricultural use. Water for irrigation is available from a pond and two private and a government owned tube-wells. Rice is the most important kharif crop (transplanted and broadcast) followed by jowar (big and small millets), maize, urd (black gram) sugarcane and sweet potatoes. In rabi as usual wheat is the leading crop, followed by barley, peas, gram, mustard and potatoes.

About three-fourth of the total population is Muslim, followed by 20 per cent Kurmi and Yadav and 5 per cent Harijans. About 5 per cent of the total population belongs to category A, 14 per cent of category B, rest 81 per cent falls under category C in this village. About 80 per cent of the population is non-vegetarian. Availability of calories is by and large satisfactory and fairly well in comparison to other villages. During the fieldwork the writer observed that the village community has a fair supply of cereals so as to enable them to get two square meals. But their diets lack is essential nutrients. One-tenth of the population thus is exposed to deficiency diseases and 1.23 per cent died owing to prolonged deficiency of essential nutrients. Table 5.11 serves as an index for measuring the health conditions of the village population. The figures with (-) signs indicate a tendency towards ill-health and deficiency diseases, while figures with (+) signs indicate better position in respect of essential nutrients needed for keeping good health.

Unlike other villages here too caloric intake varies from category to category. It is evident from Table 5.11 that the intake of calories per head day in category (A) is about 2545.4 whereas it is 2349.4 and 2163.3 in categories (B) and (C) respectively. Supply of other nutrients are also not uniformly distributed among the villagers belonging to different income groups, e.g. the position of protein and fat is good in category A but it is in short supply in categories B and C (–3.2, –7.2 and –9.3, –35.1 per cent). Supply of iron is fairly high in all the categories whereas the availability of carbohydrates, calcium, vitamin-A and vitamin-C has registered its shortage among the rural community. These nutrients are short to the level of –4.5, –38.7, –31.8 and –44.4 per cent, in the case of category A, whereas in the other two categories (B) and (C), it falls short to the level of –12.0, –44.2, –46.1, –27.6 and –7.3, –53.0, –59.6, –40.6 per cent respectively. Other nutrients, e.g. thiamine, riboflavin and niacin have registered a good supply in the first two categories. Riboflavin, however, is short

Table 5.11 : Sonbarsa : Supply of Different Nutrients per head per day in the Categories A, B, C, and percentage of Departure from Standard Requirement

Elements of Food	*Standard Requirement*	*Actual Intake* A	*Actual Intake* B	*Actual Intake* C	*PDSR* A	*PDSR* B	*PDSR* C
Protein g	68	75.9	65.85	61.7	+11.6	-3.2	-9.3
Fat g	50	61.7	46.4	32.5	+23.4	-7.2	-35.1
Carbohydrate g	440	420.3	385.6	407.7	- 4.5	-12.0	-7.3
Calcium mg	700	428.8	390.5	328.8	- 38.7	-44.2	- 53.0
Iron mg	22.5	49.48	4.31	36.5	+119.9	+91.5	+62.2
Vitamin-A I.U.	3500	2386.4	1886.8	1412.3	-31.8	-46.1	-59.6
Thiamine mg	1.12	2.36	2.0	1.94	+110.7	+78.6	+73.2
Riboflavin mg	1.46	1.65	2.01	1.14	+13.0	+37.6	-21.9
Niacin mg	19	20.1	28.19	20.7	+5.8	+48.4	+9.1
Vitamin-C mg	43	23.9	31.11	25.5	-44.4	-27.6	-40.6
Calories	2400	2545.4	2349.3	2163.3	+6.1	-2.1	-9.9

b y

–21.9 per cent in category C, while the other two vitamins are fairly well in this category too.

Deficiency of essential nutrients weekens the resistance against the diseases. Consequently, a number of deficiency diseases are prevalent in the this village but the mortality rate is comparatively low being only 1.23 per cent. The obvious reason for low rate of mortality lies in the fact that it is a small village and its cleanliness poses no problem for the rural population. Further the houses are kept free from dampness and bad smell. Other factors that contribute to the higher rate of mortality are also to a large extent non-existant.

Deficiency of protein, calories, fat, calcium and vitamin-A has caused 9.7, 13.2, 8.4, 18.1 per cent of the deficiency patients to suffer from kwashiorkor/marasmus, rickets, ostomalasia, and eye diseases (night and colour blindness, xerophthalmia, keratomalacin) etc. and several other inflammations (Fig. 5.9).

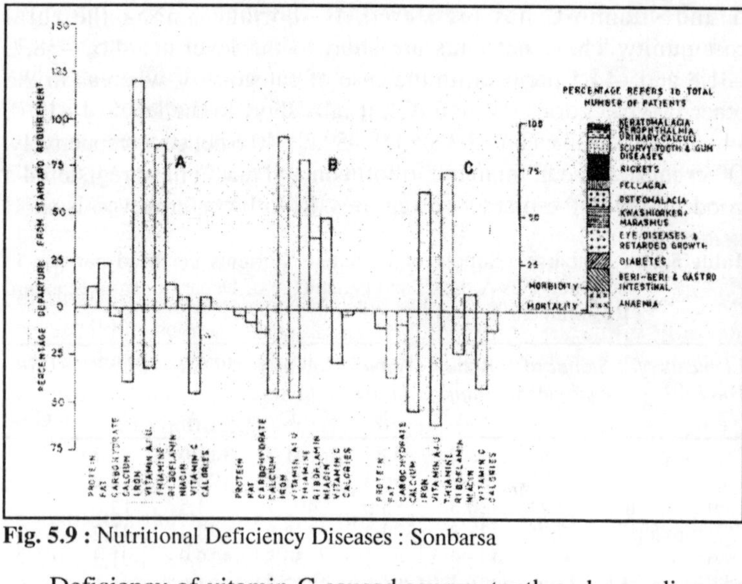

Fig. 5.9 : Nutritional Deficiency Diseases : Sonbarsa

Deficiency of vitamin-C caused scurvy, tooth and gum diseases and accounted for 6.6 per cent, the lowest in all the twelve villages under study. Apart from these diseases anaemia, beri-beri, diabetes, pellagra and urinary calculi is also found in the village and accounts for 12.2, 11.8, 8.1, 5.6 and 4.3 per cent respectively. Anaemia does exist specially in females and children although iron intake is in surplus but the deficiency of vitamin-C and other reasons discussed earlier give way to such problems. Same may be said to be the reason for cases of beri-beri, pellagra as the elements of thiamine, niacin and by and large riboflavin is fairly supplied.

It would, therefore, be correct to say that the villagers are exposed to multi-nutrients deficiency, worse among them are the low income category people, who represent a majority of population. They suffer from the deficiency of multiple nutrients at a time.

Unchegaon

The village of Unchegaon is located at a distance of approximately 5 km north of Gosaigunj town and 12 km west of tahsil Tanda. It lies 26°37′55″ north latitude and 82°42′20″ east longtitude in the district Faizabad.

Unchegaon is not favourably situated from the view point of accessibility. There is no metalled road connecting it with any neighbouring town. However, there is one partly metalled and partly *kankar* (unmetalled) road which runs to the north of the village at a distance of 1.5 km in the east-west direction. During the rainy season, this road also becomes unserviceable and another unmetalled road which comes from Gosaigung becomes almost unserviceable due to water logging. Mahboobgunj is the nearest market town 1.5 km away for day-to-day necessities.

Unchegaon lies in a level plain which has fairly good drainage and protected from the ravages of floods and also enjoys facilities of irrigation through nearby canal and tube-wells, wells etc. High percentage of cultivated land is irrigated in both the seasons. Good irrigation coupled with high yielding variety seeds, fertilizing good quality land makes the agriculture profitable and easy to make full utilization of the land. Often farmers take three crops in a year. Among the cereal crops, rice comes first, followed by wheat and pulses. Under cash crops, sugarcane comes first, then comes potato, melons and sugarbeets, course grains like maize and some small millets are also grown. On the whole, the village is agriculturally rich. A good portion of land is also devoted to mango groves and guava which give good returns to the owners. The population of the village is 1482 (2001) consisting of 432 males and 437 females and 613 children, belonging to Muslims, Hindus with majority of scheduled castes, i.e. Harijan and Pasis.

Muslims are the influential group and hold a very high portion of land. By and large, the village is non-vegetarian and enjoys an excellent position in terms of protein, fat, calcium, iron, vitamin-A etc. except carbohydrate and vitamin-C in the families of (A) category per head per day but this position does not occur in the case of (B) and (C) categories. However, this position is better in comparison to the other villages. It is clear from the Table 5.12 that on the whole, the inhabitants are well-fed. Agriculture is the main occupation of the rural communities but at least 25 per cent of the total adults are working outside the village. Thus 75 per cent will be directly dependents on agriculture; higher percentage of outside earners are from category (A) and (B).

Table 5.12 : Unchegaon : Supply of Different Nutrients per head per day in the Categories A, B, C, and percentage of Departure from Standard Requirement.

Elements of Food	*Standard Requirement*	*Actual Intake* A	*Actual Intake* B	*Actual Intake* C	*PDSR* A	*PDSR* B	*PDSR* C
Protein g	68	80.6	63.4	48.9	+18.5	-6.8	-28.1
Fat g	50	55.7	36.8	19.2	+11.4	-26.4	-61.6
Carbohydrate g	440	410.6	429.2	371.1	-6.7	-2.5	-15.6
Calcium mg	700	1337.5	1070.0	555.0	+91.1	+52.8	- 20.7
Iron mg	22.5	59.2	41.6	31.6	+160.0	+84.8	+40.4
Vitamin-A I.U.	3500	4809.0	2672.1	1787.0	+37.4	-23.6	-48.9
Thiamine mg	1.12	2.0	1.82	1.48	+63.9	+49.2	+21.3
Riboflavin mg	1.46	2.2	1.79	1.16	+50.6	+22.6	-20.5
Niacin mg	19	24.6	17.3	12.1	+29.4	-8.9	-36.3
Vitamin-C mg	43	36.3	29.2	18.8	-15.5	-23.1	-56.3
Calories	2400	2502.9	2361.0	2133.0	+4.2	-1.6	-11.1

There is very little variation in the intake of calories among the villagers belonging to different communities but this variation is not very much, viz. 2503 in A, 2361 in B and 2133 in C categories. However, the variation in case of protein, fat, calcium, vitamin-A and riboflavin is remarkably different in A from those of B and C. All the five nutrients are supplied in plenty in category A, +18.5, +11.4, +91.1, +37.4 and +50.6 per cent which seem to be quite rare in other villages irrespective of their categories. As mentioned earlier, category (A) consists of generally non-vegetarian rich people who use meaṭ, 'ghee', milk regularly. Whereas supply of these nutrients among the people of (B) category excluding calcium and riboflavin +52.8, +22.6, respectively the rest, viz. protein, fat, vitamin-A are short to the tune of –6.8, 26.4 and vitamin A –23.6. Carbohydrates are almost evenly distributed among the villagers and are only short by –6.7 (A), –2.5 (B) and –15.6 (C) per cent respectively. Supply of iron and thiamine is fairly in surplus in all categories + 160 (A), 84.8 (B), +40.4 (C) per cent and +63.9, +49.2, + 21.3 respectively whereas vitamin-C (Ascorbic acid) is short supplied in the whole village –15.5 (A) –23.1 and –56.3 per cent but it supply varies with the intake of seasonal fruits, like mango in the summer season when its supply is fairly good. Niacin is recorded in surplus only in A category +29.4 but in B and C it is short to the tune of –8.9 and –36.3 per cent. People in (C) category do not enjoy the recommended amount of protein, fat, vitamin-A and riboflavin, rather they get to the tune of –28.1, –61.6, –48.9 and –20.5 per cent respectively.

A detailed analysis of nutritional position of the village is shown in Table 5.12 prepared on the basis of data regarding their foods consumed in a week's time in three different seasons. These three tables show the per head per day intake of different essential nutrients in the different economic groups i.e. A, B, C, together with the standard requirement and their percentage departure from the given standard (PDSR). Also simultaneously disease survey was undertaken to record the morbidity and mortality rate in the village and the patients under deficiency diseases.

Out of the total population about 8.2 per cent is suffering from various diseases, accounting for 68 per cent as deficiency patients; majority of the patients comes from (C) and (B) categories where the supply is inadequate as compared to (A). This imbalance has ultimately led to the spread of several deficiency diseases (Fig. 5.10), beri-beri, and gastrointestinal disturbances, rickets, together with tooth and gum diseases scurvy accounted for more than 40 per cent of the patients. Due to deficiency of ascorbic acid, vitamin (C) riboflavin and niacin (16.8, 7.9 and 20.7 per cent respectively) vitamin-A has got a very important role in protecting people from eye diseases as well as from dry beri-beri. Its deficient supply has created several problems for human health. Its short supply in the last two categories resulted in 11.1 per cent patients suffering from various vitamin-A deficiency diseases like, nightblindness, retarded growth, xerophthalmia. Its deficiency with fat and calcium causes urinary calculi (3.2 per cent) although the supply of calcium is not short yet its mal-absorption may have helped in these diseases.

Besides these deficiency diseases, there are colitis, pellagra and marasmus. Which are caused due to the deficiency of thiamine, riboflavin, niacin and calories. The supply of these elements are not so deficient, but the absence of other essential nutrients checks its proper utilization in the body and leads to constipation, anorexia, nervus irritability, depression. The prolonged deficiency of these nutrients helped the causation of pellagra (12.2 per cent) and marasmus. Supply of protein, calories are also not satisfactory among B and C categories of people with the result that about 10.6 per cent of the total deficiency patients in the village suffered from kwashiorkor/ marasmus (Fig. 5.10).

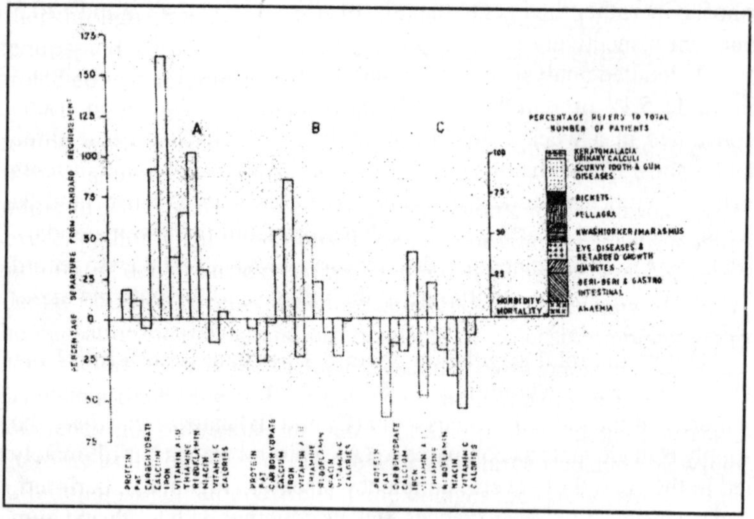

Fig. 5.10 : Nutritional Deficiency Diseases : Unchegaon

Cases of anaemia and diabetes, also exist but the number of patients suffering from these are about 9.2, 8.3 per cent respectively. Vitamin-D is scantly distributed in the villages with the result that some of them are prone to specific diseases caused due to deficient intake of vitamin-D; its shortage checks the absorption of phosphorus also. It should be kept in mind that no one nutrient functions alone and its usefulness to the body may be curtailed by the absence of other nutrients, and as only a few nutrients are stored in the body without being used because other essential nutrients are lacking in the diet.[19]

REFERENCES

1. Categories A, B and C have been formed on the basis of economic conditions determined by the size of holdings, type of land, rate of productivity, extra income and the number of family members. A, refers to such villagers whose total monthly income is above Rs. 1500; B, refers to those which fall between Rs. 800-1500 and C, represents under Rs. 800 monthly income per head of the village population.
2. Nutritive value of the different foods and their standard requirements have been calculated with the help of the table given in "The nutritive value of Indian foods and planning of a satisfactory diet" by Aykroyd, W.R. (I.C.M.R., New Delhi, 1962), and Nutritive value of Indian foods by Gopalan, C. *et al.*, Hyderabad 1977.
3. Goitre: Enlargement of thyroid glands due to long term deficiency of iodine.
4. Scurvy: Vitamin-C deficiency characterized by great debility, anaemia, mental apathy, spongy conditions of the gums and tendency to hemorrhages into the subcutaneous tissues and from the mucasis surfaces.
5. Beri-Beri: Produced by the too excessive use of polished rice, white meal flour and certain other carbohydrate staples. Characterised by degenerative changes in the nervous system including a multiple perépheral neuritis, which may exist alone (dry beri-beri), but often it combined with generalized edema and serious effusions (wet beri-beri) and by tendency to cardiac failure. Dry beri-beri is associated with the complicated deficiency of thiamine, B-complex with A and E characterized by swelling in limbs and trunk. While wet is due to thiamine deficiency alone. It is common in rice eating regions.
6. Night-Blindness: Inability to see in dim light especially when suddenly exposed to bright light.
7. Keratomalacia: Softening of the cornea, as the result of severe deficiency of vitamin-A in the body.
8. Xerophthalmia: Failure of the tear glands, followed often by dryness, bacterial growth and ulceration of cornea.
9. Pellagra: Primarily due to specific deficiency and manifests itself in symptoms affecting chiefly the skin, the elementary track and the nervous system followed by depression, dermatitis and diarrhoea.
10. Rickets: Characterised by disturbed metabolism, an impaired nutrition of the entire body and attraction in the growing bones, highest percentage of occurrence between November-May.

11. Davis, A., '*Vitality through Planned Nutrition*', New York, 1954, p. 235.
12. Srikantia, S.G., 'Anaemia and the Fortified Salt', *Hindustan Times*, New Delhi, August 4, 1975, p. 8.

13. Kwashiorkor: It is confined to children, especially upto five years of age, characterized by a subnormal weight, mental apathy, muscular wasting, changes in hair and skin pigments, followed by fatty liver, respiratory infections etc.

14. Rao, K.R., (1974) 'Nutritive Value of Protein', *Science Reporter*, May 1974, CSIR, New Delhi, p. 436.
15. Kassirsky, I., (1969) *Diseases of Warm Land* Moscow, Plotnikov, N. p. 486.

16. Nutrition Canada, National Survey, Department of National Health and Welfare, Ottawa, Canada 1973, p. 41.
17. Cardiovascular Diseases: Pertaining to Involving Heart and Blood Vessels.
18. Shafi, M., *Land Utilization in Eastern Uttar Pradesh*, 1960, p. 222.
19. Stevenson, G.T. and Miller, C., *Introduction to Food and Nutrition*, New York, 1960.

6 Summary, Conclusion and Suggestions

The Central Ganga-Ghaghra Doab comprising the districts, of Faizabad, Ambedkar Nagar and Sultanpur, consists of altogether 5335 villages. Hence it is not possible for an individual to survey all these villages, because this will involve heavy expenditure and require a number of years to complete the project. The area under study, on the whole, presents homogeneous conditions with regard to environmental conditions, pattern of agricultural products, economic level of the rural community and their dietary habits. In view of these facts, the present study spread over 12 villages may be considered valid to a large extent to arrive at a reasonable conclusion in respect of the prevalence of deficiency diseases in the rural communities of the area.

The area under study is primarily an agricultural one, where about 80 per cent of the inhabitants are engaged in agricultural pursuits. Their activities are to a large extent controlled by physical environment, e.g. climate, relief, drainage and soil. These factors together result in the production of different crops, cereals and non-cereals which provide the source of livelihood for the rural population. Besides the supply of grains, vegetables are also easily available for consumption. Milk and milk products, meat, fish and fruits are consumed by the villagers on a restricted scale due to many reasons. Therefore, the village community is by and large has to depend mostly on cereals, pulses and vegetables for their daily diets.

The study of the selected villages shows that the pressure of population on the land is considerably high. Although the percentage of the cultivated land is also high, nevertheless in each case some amount of cultivated land remains unproductive owing to various factors, i.e. injurious salts or high percentage of sand. The percentage of unproductive land is greater in the agriculturally/economically backward villages, situated in the ill-drained plain. Here, the main cause of its occurrence is due to water-logging and relatively high water table which in villages like Mumtaznagar, a good portion of land is useless due to depression infested with weeds and soil erosion renders the land unproductive. In order to check the extension of waste land, it is essential to bring improvement in the drainage system with a view to provide water to the rice fields or the water so stored may be utilized in the winter season. Besides this, the improvement will also be helpful in protecting the enormous quantity or combined nitrogen which lies in the pore space of soil. The soil texture would improve and would thus lead to better utilization of the existing cultivated land. In both the agricultural seasons the cultivated land is dominated by the grain crops. The major summer crops are rice, jowar, maize and sugarcane. Potatoes and sweet potatoes are sown as cash crops. Wheat mixed with barley and peas dominate the land in the winter season. The net-cropped land, in both the seasons are almost equal as in the summer, some crops continue till the winter season and at the same time some of the land is left fallow in the summer season to regain fertility for the winter season.

The occupational structure of the village population shows that agriculture is the main occupation of the majority of the rural communities. In every village more than 70 per cent of the population is exclusively dependent on the cultivation of land. The remaining population mostly serves the primary rural population through ancillary services and thus indirectly depends on land. However a small percentage finds some means of livelihood in the close by cities and towns.

In the area under study as well as in other parts of rural India, percentage of literacy is very low and a high percentage of the population is poor. In such circumstances, the rural population finds itself in a helpless position. Because of illiteracy, most of the villagers do not understand the implications of under and mal-nutrition and on account of unstable economic conditions, they cannot afford to take nutritive diets. Besides these factors, some of them are tied down to their traditional food habits. Religious and cultural factors too contribute to the mal-adjusted dietary habits. Finally, as revealed by the survey, most of the people do not bother or do not try to understand these terms—nutrition and balanced diet. They eat food to satisfy their hunger. They know that certain food tastes good but they could not afford to have it. Their desire to have certain food items is not because of its nutritive value but because of its taste. Food habits are generally related to types of food products available to the villagers under the existing geographical environments. Most of them are ignorant about the nutritive value of the daily diets. Some of the nutritional diseases, e.g. endemic goitre, dental carries and fluorosis having their connection with environmental factors. A survey relating to morbidity and mortality conducted in the villages has disclosed the environmental factors involved in order to control or restrict their harmful effects on human health. Changes in the environmental factors, if made within certain limits, do not produce abnormalities in the body functions. But when exposed to stress, adaptability may be impaired, body becomes vulnerable, more liable to develop disease in extreme cases. The lack of exposure of the patient to the Sun is not due to bad weather conditions but because of religions and social customs prevailing in these areas, which force some of the women folk to stay indoor or cover their entire bodies while going out of their houses. The main incidence of osteomalacia is among the child bearing women who are sometimes immobilized by their spouses and who may need a care for support in walking.

The occurrence of the deficiency disease is the result of long term and under mal-nutrition. This may be ascribed to either low production of nutritive food stuff or short supply of essential elements of food available from the individual farms. Even with normal harvest, nearly half of the population live on less than 1600 calories per head per day and consequently a partial failure of crops, reduce the diets of many poor persons to disastrously low level. In either case, the result is that people start developing various nutritional deficiency diseases. As this situation remains almost static, deficiency disease becomes a permanent feature in the rural areas of the country. However, deficiency of a single nutrient may not lead to any particular disease but in combination with other essential nutrients may prove an effective instrument in the causation of deficiency diseases. Varying degree of deficiency of nutrients, the extent to which human body can resist in variable climatic conditions is an important factor which determines the nature and degree of deficiency diseases. No one nutrient functions alone and its usefulness to the body may be curtailed by the absence of other nutrients and as only a few nutrients are stored in the body, some nutrients may be discarded by the body without being used because other essential nutrients are lacking in the diet.[1] Fat is the carrier of vitamin-A, B_6 (pyridoxin), D, E and K and helps in calcium absorption, when no fat or less fat is given, calcium is lost by the large intestine.[2] Proteins also seek cooperation of certain vitamins and their lack results in abnormal intermediary reactions of amino-acids and formation of unusual and often deleterious products, while a number of vitamins appeared to have specific roles in protein metabolism.[3] It is also said that the diets that are markedly deficient in one vitamin are often low in others too[4] or in other words supply of energy for the muscle and other tissue-function which goes all the time and ensure a supply of all the nutrients and vitamins and minerals needed to regulate and control the complicated metabolic process of the body, the effects of all vitamins overlap and interlace to such a degree that no disease is caused by any single vitamin deficiency.

The rate of occurrence of deficiency diseases among the villagers is higher where the nutritional intake is lower. The villages placed in a better position with regard to caloric intake, protein etc., though not free from such problems yet are not so severely affected. The author has noticed that the villages which are agriculturally prosperous or with better agricultural efficiency have better distribution in comparison to the non-prosperous villages, which recorded low caloric intake. With a single exception of village Gaura-Baremau (agriculturally/economically prosperous) which has lower caloric intake in comparison to the village Jhakha-Sheopur which is agriculturally/economically non-prosperous.

There is no village understudy where the mortality rate is nil, it does vary from village to village, as the rate of morbidity is different from each other.

Approximately 60 per cent of the farming community of the twelve villages is vegetarian and most of them cannot afford to consume milk products as part of their daily diets. Further, it is also clear from the available data that there is close relationship between per capita income of the villager and the caloric intake per head per day. In the village Sonbarsa, where the per capita income is highest among the villages studied, the daily caloric intake comes to about 2352 only –2 per cent short of standard requirement of 2400 per head per day, while in Mumtaznagar, where the soil is poor and production of crops depends upon the mercy of flood-causing river, the average caloric intake per head per day is only 2043, short by –14.7 per cent. The reason for lower caloric intake may be ascribed to the lower production and thereby lower per capita consumption. It is obvious from Table 6.1 that the average caloric intake varies from 2043 to 2352[5] per head per day in the twelve villages understudy whereas the average intake of these twelve villages comes to 2211.2[6] which is short by 7.9 per cent in comparison with the standard requirement of 2400 per head per day, given by ICMR after talking into consideration all groups of people, nature of their work and age etc.[7] L.D. Stamp has recommended 2460 calories per head per day for north-western Europe[8] but that area is different in climate and agricultural practice. But M. Shafi has suggested for Eastern Uttar Pradesh that an actual intake of 2000 calories per head per day is adequate.[9] Comparing these norms prescribed by different writers with the available number of calories in the villagers surveyed by the author, it has been found that the average daily intake is satisfactory throughout the villagers if tested on 2000 level but if tested on 2400 level which is recommended level, all the villages registered shortages, none has more than –14.7 per cent. Taking into consideration the actual intake as mentioned for villages especially in lower starta (category C), it is far below any standard recommendation. However, daily caloric intake is not always an index for a normal health. The other factors like mal- and under-nutrition are much more important, because a person taking required number of calories may suffer from deficiency diseases if daily diets lack essential nutrients. Summary Table 6.1 indicates the average surplus and deficient supply of various nutrients like protein, fat, carbohydrates, calcium, vitamin-A, riboflavin and vitamin-C (ascorbid acid) are usually in deficient supply and lead to severe health problem in the rural areas. Further, the average supply of iron, thiamine and to some extent niacin are distributed well above the recommended requirement in all the twelve villages but certainly not in all the economic categories except iron. The rural communities mostly being vegetarian as their diets generally based on cereals, pulses, vegetables and *gur* (raw sugar), are more deficient in comparison to their counterparts who can take more nourishing diets.

It is obvious from Table 6.1 that the supply of essential nutrients is not satisfactory in any of the twelve villages understudy. The average supply of three nutrients, e.g. fat, vitamin-A and calories are deficient in all the villages, whereas protein, carbohydrates and calcium are short supplied in nine villages and vitamin-C in ten villages at varying degrees. Riboflavin and niacin are also deficient in some of the villages. All the villages except Dhanipur, Jhakha-Sheopur, Kichaucha and Khizrabad, experience deficient supply of riboflavin, while niacin is short only in Jhakha-Sheopur and Unchegaon. Average intake of iron and thiamine is surplus in all the villages.

Table 6.1 : Average Supply of Different Nutrients and Percentage of Departure from Standard Requirement

Foed	Protein Gms		Fat Gms		Carbohydrates Gms		Calcium Mg		Iron Mg		Vitamin-A I.U.		Thiamine Mg.		Riboflavin Mg.		Niacin Mg.		Vitamin-C Mg.		Calories	
Standard	68		50		440		700		22.5		3500		1.12		1.46		19		43		2400	
	AAI	PDSR	AAI	PDSR	AAI	PDSR	AAI	PDSR	AAI	PDSR	AAI	PDSR	AAI	PDSR	AAI	PDSR	AAI	PDSR	AAI	PDSR	AAI	PDSR
Mumtaz nagar A	48.5	-23.9	23.6	-52.7	461.4	+4.9	427.8	-38.8	53.9	+139.1	1627.5	-53.5	2.1	+87.5	1.48	+1.37	19.91	+4.5	15.4	-63.0	2043.7	-14.7
Mullathi Brasin	49.9	26.7	18.7	-62.5	468.7	+6.5	453.6	-35.2	43.3	+92.7	2570.7	-26.6	1.68	+50.0	1.61	+10.3	19.7	+3.7	19.15	-55.5	2134.0	-11.1
Dhanipur A	60.1	-11.6	44.2	-11.8	370.2	-15.9	376.8	-46.2	43.2	+92.0	1693.2	-51.6	2.07	+84.8	1.32	9.6	23.7	+24.7	25.2	-41.4	2132.3	-11.2
Jhakha Sheopur	45.9	-32.5	30.5	-39.0	449.4	+2.1	582.8	-16.7	40.9	+97.8	2295.6	-34.4	1.61	+43.8	1.40	-4.1	17.8	-6.3	-26.4	38.6	2215.6	-7.7
Kichaucha	69.4	+2.1	48.8	-2.4	397.4	-9.7	1002.1	+43.1	32.9	+46.3	2860.2	-18.3	1.73	+54.5	1.29	-11.64	21.2	+11.6	32.3	-24.9	2104.8	-12.33
Khizrabad	62.8	-7.6	28.8	-42.4	397.4	-9.7	785.4	+12.2	39.4	+75.2	2526.8	-27.8	1.73	+54.5	1.29	-11.6	20.1	+5.8	29.0	-32.5	2101.5	-12.3
Ariya	71.8	+5.5	41.7	-16.7	427.7	-2.8	696.2	-0.54	53.1	+136.9	2117.2	-39.5	1.68	+50.0	1.55	+6.2	20.1	+5.8	33.3	-22.6	2343.3	-2.4
Dashrathpur	67.4	-0.9	41.8	-16.4	425.3	-3.3	400.3	-42.8	51.2	+127.7	2783.9	-20.5	1.94	+73.2	1.49	+2.1	20.0	+5.3	36.4	-15.3	2315.0	-3.5
Gaura Baremau	71.33	+4.9	35.7	-28.5	405.8	-7.8	397.2	-43.3	45.2	+100.9	3466.4	-0.96	2.26	+96.0	1.99	+36.7	19.4	+2.3	46.3	+7.7	2190.0	-8.7
Ramnathpur	62.5	-8.1	37.4	-25.3	415.8	-5.5	437.0	-37.6	49.8	+121.2	3487.4	-0.36	1.96	+75.0	1.5	+2.7	19.7	+3.7	65.9	+53.3	2265.7	-5.6
Sonbarsa	67.8	-0.29	46.8	-6.4	404.5	-8.1	382.7	-45.3	43.0	+91.3	1895.2	-45.9	2.1	+87.5	1.6	+9.6	+20.9	+20.5	26.8	-37.7	2352.7	-2.0
Unchegaon	64.3	-5.4	37.3	-25.4	403.6	-8.3	987.5	+41.1	44.1	+96.0	3089.3	-11.7	1.76	+64.0	1.95	+33.7	18.0	-5.3	28.1	-34.7	2332.3	-2.8

A Represents Economically Backward Villages
B Economically Prosperous Villages
AAI Actual Average Intake
PDSR Percentage departure from the standard requirement
\+ Indicates the surplus supply of particular element of diet among the village community
\- Indicates the deficiency supply of particular element of diet among the village community

There is a close relationship between the mal-nutrition and the deficiency diseases prevalent among the villagers. It can be argued that the village having better supply of nutrients has lesser morbidity and mortality rates in comparison to villages experiencing worst position in respect of nutritive diets (Table 6.2). Unchegaon is the village having better position in terms of intake of nutrients with the result that only 0.8 per cent of the patients died of deficiency diseases, while in the villages of Jhakha-Sheopur and Mumtaznagar with 14.6 and 14.2 per cent morbidity rates registered 1.7 per cent and 2.7 per cent deaths on account of deficiency disease respectively.

Main deficiency diseases from which the area suffers are anaemia, beri-beri and gastrointestinal disturbances, diabetes, eye diseases (night and colour blindness, xerophtalmia, keratomalacia, retarded and stunted growth, goiter, kwashiorkor/marasmus, osteomalacia, pellagra, rickets, scurvy/tooth and gum diseases and urinary calculi. It has been noticed during the survey that the maximum cases of such diseases are from lower income group (category C); these people are more prone to such diseases than the people of the other two groups (A and B).

A prolonged short supply of five essential nutrients, i.e. protein, fat, calcium, vitamin-A and C, among the rural communities has caused heavy damage to their health. They have become easy victim of kwashiorkor/marasmus (protein caloric shortage), eye diseases and related problems, osteomalacia, urinary calculi, rickets, scurvy/tooth and gum diseases. It is clear from Table 6.2 that the number of patients who suffered from, beri-beri, eye diseases, rickets and scurvy along with tooth and gum diseases are greater than those who suffered from anaemia, kwashiorkor/marsmus, pellagra etc. It is also evident from the same table that the highest morbidity rate has been found in Jhakha-Sheopur, i.e. 14.6 per cent and lowest in the village Unchegaon, with 8.2 per cent, whereas the mortality rate of 2.7 per cent in the village Mumtaz Nagar is the highest among the twelve villages and the lowest is reported from the villages Unchegaon with 0.8 per cent.

Goitre is not killing disease. It is commonly found in this area and particulary in the village Mumtaznagar, about 13.5 per cent of the deficiency patients suffered from this disease, which resulted in physical disability. This is an endemic disease in the areas of the terai where drinking water lacks iodine and the crops grown with such water also lacks iodine contents. Such cases are reported from other four villages too but their percentage share is very low. Apart from

Table 6.2 : Percentage Prevalence of Deficiency Diseases, Morbidity and Mortality Rate

Name of the Village	Morbidity Rate	Mortality Rate	Anaemia	Beri-Beri and Gastrointestinal Colities	Diabetes	Eye Diseases Stunted Retarded Growth	Goitre	Kwashiorkor/ Marasmus	Osteo-malacia	Pellagra	Rickets	Scurvy Tooth and Gum Diseases	Urinary Calculi	Xeroph-thalmia	Kerato-malacia
1	2	3	4	5	6	7	8	9	10	11	12	13	14	15	16
Mumtaznagar	14.2	2.7	10.2	15.6	8.2	9.2	13.5	5.5	2.4	3.7	14.2	13.7	1.3	-	2.5
Mullathi - Barasin	13.6	1.9	11.9	12.2	5.1	13.5	-	9.7	2.1	14.2	7.3	19.3	2.3	2.4	-
Dhanipur	12.3	1.6	13.8	14.9	1.5	16.3	2.5	7.1	4.6	3.1	15.7	15.9	3.1	1.5	-
Jhakha - Sheopur	14.6	1.7	13.1	16.2	4.0	15.6	-	6.9	6.5	7.2	10.4	17.4	2.7	-	-
Kichaucha	11.8	1.4	9.9	16.4	3.3	10.9	1.9	6.7	4.2	12.2	6.8	18.6	7.1	-	2
Khizrabad	12.7	1.9	12.8	15.6	2.5	17.9	-	11.5	3.2	8.1	12.8	11.6	4.0	-	-
Ariya	10.5	1.4	11.5	14.6	4.8	12.8	1.5	7.6	3.5	6.8	19.2	16.1	6.1	3.0	2.5
Dashrathpur	9.6	1.0	10.9	16.1	4.5	12.3	-	9.9	4.9	8.1	11.7	14.0	5.6	2.0	-
Gaura - Baremau	9.0	1.6	12.2	13.5	6.4	10.6	-	10.8	4.6	9.2	12.5	13.1	4.1	1.5	1.5
Ramnathpur	11.8	1.5	10.6	12.7	4.6	10.2	3.6	12.2	6.5	9.8	11.3	11.6	6.9	-	-
Sonbarsa	11.4	1.2	12.2	11.8	8.1	15.1	-	9.7	8.4	5.6	13.2	6.6	4.3	2.0	1.0
Unchegaon	8.2	0.8	9.2	16.8	8.3	10.1	-	10.6	-	12.2	7.9	20.7	3.2	-	1.0

goitre, there are a few more diseases which are not reported from every village, i.e. osteomalacia, xerophthalmia and keratomalacia.

Unhygienic living conditions with faulty dietary habits lead to higher morbidity. The rate is also affected by seasonal and climatic changes, e.g. hot moist weather conditions suits intestinal infections, whereas eye diseases are more common during hot weather conditions. Apart from the water pollution, air pollution and food contamination are indeed other problems. Water supply in the villages are from the open wells or from the nearby ponds, which may be easily polluted. If the villagers are provided with deeply sunk hand pumps, they will not only be free from polluted water but instead they may get some lodin. This will help in protecting the against the thyroid enlargement (goitre).

The century old system of disposal of wastes is unscientific. Latrines are constructed on the basis of old traditions, which are located within the enclosure of main residential areas and are usually without roofs, with the result that they become the breeding places for flies which may serve as the means for the spread of various infectious diseases. The habits of going to open fields answering the call of nature lead to soil pollution as well as underground water, resulting in contamination of drinking water and also cause diseases to the people moving bare-footed. Every such infection reduces the utility of vitamin-C and also causes wastage of iron etc.

The food, that human being takes is closely related to the economic condition of the rural communities. The survey conducted by the author reveals a grim situation. It is the problem of under-nutrition rather than mal-nutrition. A good percentage of rural population may often could not get two square meals a day. Some of them take only boiled gram and *gur* (raw sugar) during the day and full meal at dinner time which usually contained some cereal and pulses. This is the crux of the problem which the writer has observed in all the villages surveyed by him. The immediate problem is that everyone should get at least two meals a day and if possible, it should contain basic elements of nutrition so that the rural population could be saved from some of the deficiency diseases.

On the whole, nutritional problems are more subtle, out of sight, remote and insidious. Even when there is a enough food, there will be plenty of problems of mal-distribution (from reasons of both mal-administration and social inequality).[10]

With a better planning of lands and its products, it can be possible to improve the productivity and the standard of nutrition and health of the villagers. In India, the average yield per acre is only 1/3 to developed countries, although on the whole, it is well favoured with agricultural resources.[11] India can solve her food problems, if the people feel their responsibilities and work like Japanese, Americans, and more over it is free from natural calamities, which very often retard the overall development in the sphere of agriculture. As it has been observed that agriculturally prosperous villages show better nutritional standard, than the non-prosperous villages, it can be concluded that if agricultural productivity is increasing the fertility of the soil and making adequate arrangements for irrigation of the crops, the nutritional standard will surely improve. A detailed plan has to be chalked out for the entire area to ensure water for irrigation purposes by making reservoirs in the lowlying areas, because the erratic nature of Indian monsoons with long dry spells accompanied by high temperature is responsible for creating occasional droughts. The government should help the population in fighting the adverse effects of scarcity conditions by construction of canals, wells, tube-wells, ponds soil conservation and afforestation.

While conducting the survey the author has observed that the soil in the area under study is deficient in nitrogen protein will increase, but due to excessive use of N_2, soil becomes poor in potash and sulphate, which are essential for leguminous crops which are also rich sources of protein. The farmers tried one or two times to grow such crops but since they could not get good harvest, they dropped the idea.

Therefore, no rich protein crops are generally grown. This is the setback of hybrid variety of seeds says the farmer. However this is not true; yield may be increased by putting suitable amount of nitrogen, and organic manures coupled with proper irrigation. N_2 in combination with P_2O_2 in recommend proportion with sufficient water may result in three times high yield of sugarcane. However, there are other sources of nitrogenise manures, i.e. farm-yard manures, compost, oilseeds and oil cakes, green manuring and through rotation of crops.

The farmers should have enough knowledge to administer the fertilizers properly, as it is very difficult to give proper dose of fertilizers in the absence of detailed soil testing report relating to the area. In such cases, fertilizer may affect cells adversely. Keeping in view the economic conditions of the farming community, green manuring may be a cheap source of building soil fertility. Some suitable plants for green manuring should be tried which is grown before the sowing of kharif crops so that the same land may be used in kharif season. Secondly, cultivating leguminous crops in rotation may also increase fertility. The rotation of crops helps in crop planning and in increasing the soil fertility. Planning may also help in controlling weeds and certain crop pests and diseases. Sun-hemp (*Dhaincha*) is the most important green manuring crop; if grown in those fields which are left fallow, the fertility and productivity of the soil may considerably be increased. Weeds, pests and diseases also cause much damage to the crops. Problem of *motha* (weed) troubles much in the kharif season. It is deeply rooted and difficult to remove during ploughing. It can be minimized through deep ploughing or by leaving the land fallow or by weeding out the undesirable plants. Menace is less in clay than in sandy and sandy-laom. Because of excessive water and fertilizers favourable conditions for pests and diseases arise and to combat these problems proper treatment is required. The medicines which are generally used either supplied late or in storage gets expired and the use of such medicines after the expiry dates, resulted in poor performance with less effectiveness. Proper medicines should be given with the demonstration to use them effectively within the valid dates.

Residual effect of grain is another problem. Pesticides and chemicals used to save the grain from the rodents and other insects, affect the health of villagers by contaminating grains also. The grains when left open are contaminated by birds. So special care is to be taken in storage and to avoid contaminated grains used so that people could be saved from the ill-effects on their health.

The alarming population growth, has created problems for social and economic development of the country. Continuous increase overtakes the increase in agricultural productivity, with the result that supply of different food items cannot match the recommended requirements. The better way of keeping down the demands of food is through limitation of family size. Because of increasing prices and limited income, the availability of food to each children becomes low; not only this, housing, hygiene and other factors also may crop up. Lesser will be the children greater will be the availability of food and healthier and happier will be the family. But one thing should be kept in mind that the need for more children in downtrodden societies is to ensure that at least, couple of them will come up to the age of maturity and will be helpful in financial uplift of the family. However, this in tern is linked with the economic situation, food and public health problems. Further high pressure of population on agricultural land has resulted in the sub-division and fragmentation of holdings. The fragmented and uneconomic holdings have brought about a steady deterioration in agriculture and enhanced the poverty of the rural community. Since the introduction of consolidation schemes, at least for the time being, the evils are reduced considerably.

There is a scope for raising more yields from the land at reduced cost by using efficient farm implements. Due attention is being given in this direction and more new equipments are being introduced but not at a desired level. Because these implements cost much which the poor farmer cannot afford and also it may not be much economical seeing the size of the holdings.

The problem of rural finance should be taken care of by the government. The cultivators should be given financial assistance in time on credit to buy high yielding variety of seeds, manures and other accessories. Although the government has already taken steps in this direction yet the funds allocated are not enough; secondly, due to red-tapism, funds are not given in time or may not get the full amount requested in certain cases. It is desirable to establish a sort of pool system in every village and operate jointly where the right of every owner of land is safeguarded and recognized. This will not only enhance the yield per hectare but also pave the way for easy management of farm loans, procurement of modern agricultural equipments which will increase the agricultural production. The production can also be increased by introducing the new varieties of seeds which have been discovered by the Agricultural Research Institute (New Delhi). The 'Green Revolution' has made tremendous achievements in the sphere of agriculture and various late and early varieties of cereal and non-cereal crops are now grown with high yields.

In the opinion of the author the solution of the present problem lies not only in the increase of productivity of agricultural crops, but also in the proper distribution of the product among the rural population so as to ensure qualitatively and quantitatively adequate diet for an individual. Care should also be taken to see that the daily diets of the rural population contain essential nutrients which might be provided by cheaper food items. To reduce the conditions of under and mal-nutrition created by faulty dietary habits, it is essential to make relevant modification in the food habits of the farming community by suggesting more nutritive foods which the middle and low income group of people could afford. Further as said, a change in cropping pattern will enable the farmers to cultivate such crops which could give them some essential food nutrients, e.g. protein from pulses and vitamin-A and C and calcium through leafy vegetables.

It would not be out of place to mention here that the present problems need a more detailed study, which can be conducted by a team workers and in which geographer has to play an important role. As the present study has been made solely by a geographer, it is very much true that some important medical aspects of the various deficiency diseases could not be studied or discussed in depth.

REFERENCES

1. Stevenson, G.T. and Miller, C., *Introduction to Food and Nutrition*, New York, 1960, p. 38.
2. Davis, A., *Vitality through Planned Nutrition*, New York, 1954, pp. 30-31.
3. Wiggers, C.J., *Physiology of Health and Disease Philadelphia*, 1955, p. 918.
4. Diehl, H.S., *Healthful Living*, New York, 1964, p. 98.
5. Refers to average of categories A, B, C of the people in each village.
6. Refers to average of all the twelve villages under study.
7. Aykroyd, W.R., *The Nutritive Value of Indian Foods and Planning of a Satisfactory Diet*, New Delhi, ICMR, 1963, p. 26.
8. Stamp, L.D., *Our Developing World*, London, 1960, p. 110.
9. Shafi, M., *Land Utilization in Eastern Uttar Pradesh*, Aligarh, 1960, p. 222.
10. W.H.O., '*Nutrition*' (Neglected Factor in National Development), Delhi, 1972, p. 14.
11. Clifford, M.H., '*Over Coming World Hunger*', London, Series No. 2, 1969, p. 52.

Bibliography

Achuthan, K., *Lessons from Recurring Drought*, Swarajya, Madras, June 14, 1975.

Agarwal, R. P., *Soil Fertility in India*, Bombay, 1965.

Agarwal, S. K., The Determinants of Malnutrition in Rural Haryana, India, *Culture, Society and Economy* (eds.) Mukerji, A.B and Ahmad, Aijazuddin, Inter-India Publication, New Delhi, 1985.

Ahmad, A., *Health Care is an Indicator of Social well being* : a case study of the tribal territories in India. Abstract of Papers IGU working group on Geography of Health, Tokyo, 1980.

Ahmad, S.W., Distribution of Nutritional Deficiency Diseases in Faizabad District, *The Geographer*, Vol. XXV, No. 1, 1978.

Ahmad, S.W, Dietary Habits and Nutrition in Sultanpur District, *Geographical Outlook*, Vol. XIV, 1978-79.

Ahmad, S.W., Distribution of Pulse Protein in Uttar Pradesh, *National Geographical Journal of India*, Varanasi, 1978.

Ahmad, S.W., The Distribution of Calories, Fat and Carbohydrates Produced from Various Crops of Uttar Pradesh, The Geographer, Vol. XXVI, 1979.

Akhtar R., *Environment, Agriculture and Nutrition in Kumaon Region*, Marwah Publication, New Delhi, 1980.

Akhter, R., Environmental factors and heath in India, *Philippine Geographical Journal*, Vol. 23, No. 2, 1979.

Albrecht, W. A., *Physical, Chemical and Bio-chemical Changes in the Soil Community*, London, 1967.

Ali, Mohammad, *Food and Nutrition in India*, Rajesh Pub., Dariaganj, New Delhi, 1977.

Amar, H., *The Sociological Approach to Problems of Community Development*, Arab States Fundamental Educational Centre Sirs-et-Layyan, U.A.R., 1960.

Auden, J.B. and Roy, A.C., Report on Sodium Salt in Reh Soil in

Uttar Pradesh: Report on *Geological Survey of India*, Calcutta, 1942.

Armstrong, R. W., Cancer and Soil, *Professional Geographer*, 1965.

Armstrong,R.W., Medical Geography, an emerging specialty, *International Pathology*, Vol. 6, 1965.

Aurora, K.C., *Starvation and Mal-nutrition in India: Some Suggestion* (A) Madhya Pradesh Chronicle, April 24, 1972.

Austin, M.E., *Nutrition in Action*, New York, 1963.

Aykroyd, W.R., *Nutritive Value of Indian Foods and Planning Satisfactory Diet*, ICMR, New Delhi, 1966.

Aykroyd, W.R. and Verma, O.P., Superficial Keratitis due to Riboflavin Deficiency, *Indian Medical Gazetteer*, Delhi, 1942.

Azad, R. N., *Nutrition in the context: Food, Storage and Rising Population*, Kurukshetra, Feb. 11-13, 1975.

Baljit, S., *Benefit, Cost Analysis of the Sarda Canal System*, Bombay, 1965.

Barker, G., *Health in Independent India*, New Delhi, 1957.

Barret, F. A., *Medical Geography*, Concept and Definition in Medical Geography, Progress and Prospects (ed) Michael Pacione, Croom Helm, London, 1986.

Basu, J.K., *Soil Fertility, Indian Farming*, Vol. III, No. 5, New Delhi, 1973.

Berg, A., *Nutrition*, National Development and Planning, Cambridge, 1973.

Bicknell, F. and Prescott, F., *The Vitamins in Medicine*, London, 1953.

Brooks, C.E.P., *Climate in Every Day Life*, London, 1950.

Buck, J.L., *Land Utilization in China*, Namking, 1937.

Buck, A.L., The Study of the Geography of Diseases, *Geographical Review*, Vol. 125, 1959.

Cañon, H.C. Hopps, *Geological Study of Anaemia*, Calorado, 1971.

Chandra, P., Non-Nutritional Causes of Mal-Nutrition, *Ind., Jour. Nutri. and Dietetics*, Coimbatore 1975.

Chaubey, K., Disease of Sugar, City in Light of Environment and Nutritional Deficiency Factors, A study in Medical Geography, *Geog. Rev. of India*, Vol. 33, No. 2, 1971.

Chifford, M.H., *Over Coming World Hunger*, London, 1969.

Chitralekas, R., Poverty and level of Nutrition: Some more evidences. *The Indian Geographical Journal*, Vol. 57, No. 2, 1982.

Corwin, E.H.L., *Ecology and Health*, New York, 1949.

Dasman, R.F., *Environmental Conservation*, U.S.A., 1968.

Davis, A., *Vitality through Planned Nutrition*, New York, 1959.

Davis, A., *Let Us Eat Right to Keep Fit*, London, 1971.

Detwyler, T.R., *Man's Impact on Environment*, New York, 1921.

Diell, H.S., *Healthful Living*, New York, 1964.

Dubey, O.P. and Koley, Shyamal, Food and Nutrition in Samnapur. Sagar District (M.P.), *Geographical Review of India*, Vol. 59 No. 1, 1997.

Dubos, R. *Man, Medicine and Environment*, London, 1968.

Gandhi, M.K., *Diet and Diet Reforms*, Ahamadabad, 1949.

George, A.J., *Public Health of Salem District in Relation to Environment*, J.M.G.A., Vol. XI, Madras 1936-37.

Glennie, E.A., Gravity Enomalies in the Structure of the Earth's Crest, *Memories of Geological Survey of India*, Dehradune, Vol. 27, 1932.

Gopalan, C., *Nutrition and Development*, N.I.N, Hyderabad, 1972.

Gopalan, C., Ramashastri, B.V. and Balasubramaniyam, *Nutritive Value of Indian Foods*, N.I.N., Hyderabad,1977

Gopalan, C.,. *Nutritive value of Indian Foods*, Hyderabad, India, 1995.

Gupta, P.S. and Solasyuk, G., Economic Rationalization of India: Problems and Approach, *Census of India*, Monograph, No. 9, 1961.

Hall, H., *The Soil: An Introduction to the Scientific Study of the Growth of Crops*, London, 1956.

Hamlon, J.J., *Principles of Public Health Administration*, St. Lonis 1955.

Hazra, J., The Scope of Medical geography, *The Geographical Observer*, Vol. 13. 1967.

Heins, H.S., *Heinz Hand Book of Nutrition*, New York, 1959.

Howe, G.M., *Some Aspects of Medical Geography of U.K.*, Geographical Congress, Vol. I, Delhi, 1970.

Howe, G.M. at Phillips D.R. Medical Geography in United Kingdom (1945-82), In *Geographical Aspect of Health* (eds), N.D. McGlashan and J.R. Blunden, London. 1983.

Inderpal, *Aspects of Medical Geography*, University Studies in Geography, 1972.

Jones, K. and Moon, G., *Health, Disease and Society; A Critical Medical Geography*, London, 1987.

Kamat, S. A., Rainy Season Disease and their Prevention, Bombay *Civic Journal of India*, Vol. 22, No. 4, 1975.

Kassirsky, I.K. and Plotnikov, V., *Diseases of Warm Land*, Moscow, 1969.

Kawata, K., *Environmental Sanitation in India*, Ludhiana 1963.

Kendrew, W.G., *The Climate of the Continents*, Great Britain, 1961.

Krishnamurthy, C.S., *Mal-Nutrition in Infants and Deficiency Disease*: National Health Seminar, Madras, 1965.

Krishna, G., Regional Pattern of Surplus, Deficit Food Production in U.P., *Geographical Outlook*, Vol. 7, 1970-71.

Kruse, H.D., *Medical Evaluation of Nutritional Status*, Pub., Health Rep., Washington, D.C., Vol. 56, 1941.

Kumar, A., *Foodgrains Production in India*; *Impact of Techno-Environmental Factors*, New Delhi, 1988.

Kuppu Swami, S., Srivastava, M. and Subramaniyam, V., *Protein in Food*, I.C.M.R., New Delhi, 1952.

Laut, P., *Agricultural Geography*, Melbourne, 1968.

Learmonth, A.T.A., Chairman's Report to the Commission on Medical Geography, I.G.U. Congress, Delhi, 1968.

Learmonth, A.T.A., *Ecological Medical Geography of India and Pakistan*, I.G.U., XXXIII, No. 2, 1968.

Learmonth,A.T.A., Ecological Medical Geography, *Progress in Geography*, Vol. 7., London; 1975.

Learmonth, A., *Disease Ecology*, New York, 1988.

Lee, D.H.K., Physiology and Tropics, *Malayan Medical Journal*, Vol. 11, 1930.

Markham, S.F., *Climate and Energy of Nations*, London, 1942.

Maxim, E., Dixitt, M.C. and Mudambi, *Human Nutritions Principle and Application in India*, New Delhi, 1969.

May, J.M., *Studies in Disease Ecology*, New York, 1961.

May,J.M., *Ecology of Mal-Nutrition in the Near and Far East*, New York, 1961.

May, J.M., Medical Geography : Its Methods and Objectives, *Geog. Review*, Vol. 40, 1950.

May, J.M. and Wash, S., *Medical Geography*, I.G.S., 1952.

McKenley, E.B., *Geography of Disease*, Washington, 1935.

McGlashan, N.D., *Medical Geography*, London, 1972.

McGlashan, N.D., *Measles, Mal-Nutrition and Blindness*, I.G.U., Delhi, 1970.

Misra, R.P., *Medical Geography of India*, New Delhi, 1970.

Moore, W.G., *The Soil We Live On*, London, 1962.

Morgan, W.B. and Munton, R.J.C., *Agriculture Geography*, London, 1971.

Mottram, V.H., *Human Nutrition*, London, 1963.

Mukherjee, P.K., *Regional Sociology*, London, 1926.

Murray, M. A., *Exploratory Study in Urban Medical Geography*, A.A.A.G., Vol. 46, 1956.

Murray, M.A., *Geography of Death*, A.A.A.G., Vol. 52, 1962.

Napier, L.E. and Edward, M., Anaemia in Pregnancy in Calcutta, Ind. *J. Med. Res.*, Vol. 33, 1941.

Oldam, R.D., A *Mannual of Geology of India*, Calcutta, 1893.

Passmore, R.C., Mixed Deficiency Diseases in India, *Tr. Roy. Soc. Trop. Med. And Hyg.*, Vol. 41, 1947.

Patwardhan, V.N., Nutrition in India, *Ind. Jour. Med. Soc.*, 1962.

Rajamunikam, A.S., Crops of Trichinopoly District, *J.M.G.A.*, Vol. 8, 1953.

Ray Chowdhary, S.P. and Mukharjee, S.K., Present Position of Soil Survey of India, *Journal of Scientific and Industrial Research*, Vol. VI, Calcutta, 1947.

Rehman, J., Health and Environment, *Tibbiya College Magazine*, Aligarh, 1967-68.

Rogers, E.S., *Human Ecology and Health*, New York, 1960.

Rolleston, H. and Moncrieff, A.A., *Diet in Health and Disease*, Great Britain, 1939.

Sample, E.C., *Influence of Geographic Environment*, London, 1911.

Santanan, R., Nutrition in the Five Year Plan, *Yojana*, April 15, 1975.

Schiffers, J.J., *Healthier Living*, Sixth International Congress of Nutrition in Restrospect, New York, 1965.

Sen Chowdhary, L.K., We Need Food not Vitamins, *Economic Times*, January 25, 1975.

Shattuck, G.C., *Diseases of Tropics*, New York, 1951.

Shafi, M., Land Utilization in Eastern Uttar Pradesh, Aligarh, 1960.

Shafi, M., Food Production, Efficiency and Nutrition in India. *The Geographer*, Vol. 14, 1967.

Shrikantia, S.G., Anaemia and Fortified Salt, *Hindustan Times*, New Delhi, August 4, 1975.

Siddiqui, M.F., 'Concentration of Deficiency Diseases in Uttar Pradesh', *The Geographer*, Vol. XVIII, 1971.

Simmon, S.J., Whayne, F.T., Anderson, W.G., Horock, M.H. and Thomas, A.R., *Global Epidemiology: A Geography of Disease and Sanitation*, U.S.A.

Stannus, H.S., Pellagra and Pellagra Like Conditions in Warm Climate, *Tropical Disease Bulletin*, 1936.

Stamp, D.L., *The Geography of Life and Death*, London, 1964.

Stamp, D.L., *The Land of Britain, Its Use and Misuse*, London, 1962.

Stevenson, G.T. and Miller, C., *Introduction to Food and Nutrition*, New York, 1960.

Stine, W.A., Evolutionary Implications of Changing Nutritional Pattern in Human Population, *American Anthropologist*, 1973.

Sukhatme, P.V., *Feeding India's Growing Millions*, Bombay, 1965.

Swaminathan, M.S., Feed the People in India: An Integrated Nutrient Supply System, *Yojana*, March 15, 1975.

Syndenstricker, E., *Health and Environment*, New York, 1937.

Taylor, G.E. and Chhuttani, P.N., Nutritional Microcytic Anaemia and the Annual Protein Food, *Brit. Med. Jour.*, 1945.

Taylor, C.M. and Pye, O.F., *Foundation of Nutrition*, New York, 1966.

Tahiliani B., Vitamin-A Deficiency: A Common Cause of Blindness in India, *Caravan*, May 1, 1975.

Thomson, A.M. and Freeman, B., An Epidemic of Riboflavin Deficiency in Indian Troops, *Tr. Roy. Soc. Trop. Med. Hyg.*, Vol. 40, 1947.

Tuli, P., *Protein Deficiency and the Nutritional Programmes*, Tattler, Vol. 3, March 25, 1975.

Wadia, D.N., *Geology of India*, London, 1953.

Wadia, D.N. and Auden, J.B., Geology and Structure of Northern India, *Memoirs of Geological Survey of India*, Vol. 73, Delhi, 1939.

Wiggers, C.J., *Physiology of Health and Disease,* Philadelphia, 1955.

Wilson, S.G., *Preventive Medicine and Public Health*, New York, 1954.

Wilson, B.R., *Environmental Problems*, U.S.A., 1968.

Williams, J., Nutrition is Above Political Considerations, *Hitvada Magazine Section*, April, 1972.

Verhasselt, Y., Geography of Health in France and the Bencluy Centers. In *Geographical Aspect of Health* (eds) N.D. and J.R. Blunder, London, 1983.

Vijayaraghvan, K., *Ecological Constraints and Nutritional Status of the Community*, Nutrition, C.U.R., Hyderabad, 1974.

District Gazetteer of Sultanpur, Allahabad, 1903. 129. F.A.O., Protein, Haley, 1967.

F.A.O., *Nutrition and Working Efficiency*, Rome, 1966.

F.A.O. *Conflicting Doctrines about Soils*, Washington, 1948.

Final Settlement Report of District Faizabad, Allahabad, 1942.

Results of Diet Surveys in India, New Delhi, 1953.

I.C.M.R., The Nutritional Research Laboratories, Annual Reports 1953-1957.

Memoirs of Meteorological Department, Vol. XXXI, Part III, 1962.

Nutrition, NIN (I.C.M.R.), Hyderabad, 1973.

Nutrition Canada, National Survey, Department of National Health and Welfare', Ottawa, 1973.

Nutrition Strategy, *Indian Express*, City Edition, June 21, 1972.

Report on India's Food Crisis and Steps to Meet it Sponsored by the Ford Foundation, Government of India, New Delhi, 1959.

U.S. Department of Agriculture, *Climate and Man*, Washington, 1941.

U.N.O., Department of Social Affairs, Preliminary. Report on the World Social Situations with Reference to Standard of Living, New York, p. 180.

UNESCO, '*Water for the Affluent Cholera for the Poor Paris*, 1975.

W.H.O., *Nutrition*, Manila, 1974.

——, *Mal-Nutrition and Disease*, Switzerland, 1963.

——, *Protein Mal-Nutrition in South India*, Vol. 20, 1959.

——, *Nutrition and Disease*, Geneva, 1963.

——, Construction of World Health Organization, Geneva, 1964, Technical Report Ser. No. 570 Geneva, 1975.

——, *Environmental Health in Urban Development*, Report of WHO expert Committee Geneva, 1991.

——, *Our Planet, Our Health*, Report of the WHO Commission on Health and Environment, WHO, Geneva, 1992.

Index